UTIAN

MENOPAUSE IN
MODERN PERSPECTIVE

MENOPAUSE IN MODERN PERSPECTIVE

A Guide To Clinical Practice

Wulf H. Utian, M.B.B.Ch., Ph.D.,
M.R.C.O.G., F.A.C.O.G.

Associate Professor, Department of Reproductive Biology
Case Western Reserve University and
University Hospitals, Cleveland, Ohio

Formerly, Director, Menopause Research Clinic,
Groote Schuur Hospital and University of Cape Town,
Cape Town, South Africa

APPLETON-CENTURY-CROFTS / NEW YORK

LSOMM h 10

80 81 82 83 84 / 10 9 8 7 6 5 4 3 2 1

Prentice-Hall International, Inc., London
Prentice-Hall of Australia, Pty. Ltd., Sydney
Prentice-Hall of India Private Limited, New Delhi
Prentice-Hall of Japan, Inc., Tokyo
Prentice-Hall of Southeast Asia (Pte.) Ltd., Singapore
Whitehall Books Ltd., Wellington, New Zealand

Library of Congress Cataloging in Publication Data

Utian, Wulf H 1939-
    Menopause in modern perspective.

    Includes bibliographical references and index.
    1. Menopause.   I. Title.
RG186.S87   618.1'75   79-18435
ISBN 0-8385-6297-3

Text design: Myrna Sharp
Cover design: Susan Rich

PRINTED IN THE UNITED STATES OF AMERICA

Even Our Destiny Is Determined By The Endocrine Glands

Albert Einstein

Contents

FOREWORD

As an increasing percentage of the population grows older, there will be more emphasis on the management of problems related to older people. The menopause, which is simply the cessation of the reproductive years and the disappearance of menstrual flow, has long been written about and talked of as a mysterious and frequently bizarre event. Much of this folklore has been laid to rest, but, even among physicians, all manner of signs and symptoms in older women are attributed to the menopause.

The present monograph deals in a scholarly way with those events which characterize the menopausal years and its management. Dr. Utian has had considerable experience in the study of those hormonal events which accompany ovarian failure and these are all included. He has diligently searched the literature for those papers which will materially add to the understanding and management of these years. He has carefully evaluated the use of estrogen, which to many has appeared as a panacea over the years.

It is hoped that this book will bring to students at all levels an understanding of the menopause so that it will no longer be the climacteric that it is alluded to be, but merely a healthy, long life of three score and ten years, or even more.

A. Brian Little, M.D.
Professor and Director
Department of Obstetrics and Gynecology
University Hospitals of Cleveland and
Case Western Reserve University
School of Medicine
Cleveland, Ohio

PREFACE

The menopause is an emotional subject not only to women, but also to men and doctors. Nonetheless, the heated debate of the past five years among physicians, consumers, the pharmaceutical industry, and various governmental agencies has often gone beyond the bounds of rationality and scientific acceptability. The effect of such excesses upon medical practitioners involved in direct clinical care has been one of confusion. Physicians are often in doubt as to what, on the one hand, can be considered correct attitudes and acceptable standards for clinical practice, and what, on the other hand, can be an avenue to medical complication and potential litigation.

Over sixty years ago, Maranon, in the preface to his book *The Climacteric (The Critical Age)* wrote: "In considering the menopause, we face a curious fact. The newly graduated physician has scarcely more than a vague idea of what the state is and what it signifies in human physiology and pathology. If you turn to the literature for an amplification of these vague, general ideas, you will have a hard time finding a comprehensive and modern study of climacteric transition. . .yet the problem of the menopause comes up every day, every hour, in the professional work of every physician."[1]

Until the mid 1960s, there continued to exist in the medical literature a remarkable lack of established scientific data relating to human climacteric. During recent years much necessary information has been presented by leading specialists in the field through workshops and conferences, and in journals and texts. Invariably, however, the information has been presented in greater detail than required by those in clinical practice.

This book is intentionally single-authored to provide an overview, with consistency of thought and avoidance of subject overlap. Above all, it is designed as a clinical manual for the physician, the resident, and the interested medical student. The purpose is to clearly define climacteric and its related effects, to evaluate the current status of hormone replacement therapy, including the risks and benefits, and to provide clinical guidelines toward care of the perimenopausal patient. Perspective is given on an overcharged area of debate.

Throughout the book, the term *climacteric* is used to refer to that phase in the aging process of women marking the transition from the reproductive stage of life to the nonreproductive stage. *Menopause* refers to the final menstrual period that occurs during the climacteric. These definitions are in accordance with the consensus reached at the First International Congress on Menopause.[2]

[1]Maranon G: The Climacteric (The Critical Age). St. Louis, Mosby, 1929
[2]Utian WH, Serr D: The climacteric syndrome. In van Keep PA, Greenblatt RB, Albeaux-Fernet M (eds): Consensus on Menopause Research. Lancaster, MTP Press, 1976, p 1

A monograph of this nature involves a considerable number of work-hours, and the effort is made more productive by a supportive family and secretary. I thank Moira, Brett, and Lara for their understanding, and Barbara A. Yohey for spending her weekends and early mornings in typing the manuscript.

As is inevitable after many years of experience and involvement in one area of medical research, I have an enormous debt of gratitude to a large number of people. To my research colleagues at the Groote Schuur Hospital in Cape Town and the University Hospitals in Cleveland, and to my many associates of the "Menopause Club" around the world, I offer my thanks for sharing their experiences with me. It is my hope that this book, in surveying both old and new information, will represent a clinically useful analysis of the current literature on the subject.

MENOPAUSE IN
MODERN PERSPECTIVE

1

The Background

HISTORICAL ASPECTS

Three major milestones exist in the history of menopause. The first event was the achievement of Butenandt, a Nobel prize winner in chemistry. He succeeded in 1929 in isolating and obtaining, in pure form, a hormone from the urine of pregnant women which was eventually called estrone.[1] The second development was the publication of a book in 1966 by Robert A. Wilson, M.D., entitled *Feminine Forever*,[2] which became an instant best-seller. This book popularized a theory called "estrogen replacement treatment" or "hormone replacement therapy." The book not only resulted in the power of consumerism being brought directly into the office of physicians but also caused the physicians themselves to take sides in a fiery debate which still continues.

The third landmark was the publication of an editorial and two original articles in the *New England Journal of Medicine* of December 4, 1975 claiming an association between exogenous estrogens and endometrial cancer.[3] Among the effects of this publication were a reversal of popular opinion, and a demonstration of the fickleness of consumerism. It also brought in legal action by initiating, in the United States at least, a series of health administration inquiries. Inevitably, confusion was sown in the minds of the medical profession and the general public alike. Since the purpose of this book is to provide information and a perspective, a brief, historical survey of issues relating to the menopause is in order.

Menopause

The menopause, in various guises, was referred to in many early cultures and texts. Initially, an association was made between age and the loss of fertility. In the Bible, for example, "God said unto Abraham, as for Sarah thy wife . . . I will bless her and give thee a son also of her . . . then Abraham fell upon his face, and said in his heart, shall a child be born unto him that is an hundred years old? And shall Sarah, that is ninety years old bear?" (Gen. 17:15-18). By the sixth century A.D. the cessation of menstruation is well documented: "Menstruation does not cease before the thirty-fifth year, nor does it usually continue after the fiftieth year . . . fat women lose their periods very early . . . and whether the periods remain normal or abnormal, increase in amount or become diminished depends on the age, the season of the year, the habits, the peculiar traits of women, the nature of the foods eaten and complicating diseases."[4]

Similar descriptions of menstrual cessation and its age of onset continued for another thousand years. But it is not until the late eighteenth and early nineteenth centuries that the story is worth taking up again.

John Leake, in his 1777 book, *Chronic or Slow Diseases Peculiar to Women*,[5] obviously influenced by William Harvey's historic description of the circulatory system, made one of the first reasonable attempts to explain the etiology of menopause: "So long as the prime of life continues, together with that extraordinary natural faculty of preparing redundant blood for the service of the child; so long its circulating force will be more than equal to the slender resistance of the uterine vessels, and the menses will continue to flow; but when they become so firm and strong from the effect of age, that the current of blood, now diminished in quantity, is insufficient to force them open; then the periodical discharge will totally cease."[5]

A development from that time on was to link cessation of menstruation with all sorts of other problems, emotional and organic. Leake wrote that "At this *critical time of life* (his italics) the female sex are often visited with various diseases of the *chronic kind*."[5] He added that "Some are subject to pain and giddiness of the head, hysteric disorders, colic pains, and a female weakness . . . intolerable itching at the neck of the bladder and contiguous parts are often very troublesome to others." He observed that "Women are sometimes affected with low spirits and melancholy." Specific disease associations were also made. In 1814 John Burns stated that "the cessation of menses does of itself seem, in some cases, to excite cancer of the breast."[6]

Leake felt that "It may appear extraordinary that so many disorders should happen from a change so usual with every female," but explains it away as being due to the "many excesses introduced by luxury, and the irregularities of the passions." Indeed, he added that from such diseases "quadrupeds and other animals are entirely exempt by living comfortable to their natural feelings."[5]

Laying the blame for menopause on the "excesses of society" was to continue. In 1868, Charasse wrote that "a lady who has during the whole of her wifehood eschewed fashionable society and has lived simply, plainly, and sensibly, and who has taken plenty of outdoor exercise, will during the autumn and winter of her life reap her reward by enjoying what is the greatest earthly blessing — health."[7]

Edward Tilt was a British physician who wrote one of the first full-length books on "change of life." Some of his views from 1857 are summarized as follows:[8]

1. The change of life is eminently critical.
2. It is still safe and desirable to imitate the critical efforts of nature at this crisis, by bleeding, and by giving purgatives and sudorifics.
3. Women (at this time) should adhere to a judiciously laid down code of hygiene.
4. Women, at the change of life, are frequently affected with cancer, gout, and rheumatism.
5. Well-localized nervous affections sometimes occur at this critical epoch.

These statements reflect a tendency from the mid-nineteenth century onward for the medical literature to associate menopause with many negative sociologic features. This is best summarized in a statement by Colombat de L'Isère in a chapter on "Change of Life" in his *Treatise on the Diseases of Females* (1845):

> Compelled to yield to the power of time, women now cease to exist for the species, and henceforward live only for themselves. Their features are stamped with the impress of age, and their genital organs are sealed with the signet of sterility. . . . It is the dictate of prudence to avoid all such circumstances as might tend to awaken any erotic thoughts in the mind and reanimate a sentiment that ought rather to become extinct. . . in fine, everything calculated to cause regret for charms that are lost, and enjoyments that are ended forever.[9]

Earlier, he had stated that "She now resembles a de-throned queen, or rather a goddess whose adorers no longer frequent her shrine. Should she still retain a few courtiers, she can only attract them by the charm of her wit and the force of her talents."

Not all physicians took such a negative attitude. Borner, in 1887, stated:

> The climacteric, or so-called change of life in women, presents, without question, one of the most interesting subjects offered to the physician, and especially to the gynecologist, in the practice of his profession. The phenomena of this period are so various and changeable, that he must certainly have had a wide experience who has observed and learned to estimate them all. So ill-defined are the boundaries between the physiological and the pathological in this field of study, that it is highly desirable in the interest of our patients of the other sex, that the greatest possible light should be thrown upon this question.[10]

The narrow boundary between normal physiology and pathology has not been fully defined nearly a hundred years later. Nor have the many negative and largely unsubstantiated statements ceased to be made. These are evidenced by the following contemporary examples.

(1963) "A large percentage of women ... acquire a vapid cowlike feeling called a 'negative state.' It is a strange endogenous misery ... the world appears as though through a grey veil, and they live as docile, harmless creatures missing most of life's values."[11]

(1963) "The menopausal woman is not normal; she suffers from a deficiency disease with serious sequelae and needs treatment."[12]

(1966) "Often busy mothers or energetic careerists who are unwilling or unprepared to acknowledge the termination of the reproductive phase of their lives and the inception of a new era are thrown into considerable turmoil by this event."[13]

(1967) "Many women are leading an active and productive life when this tragedy strikes. They are still attractive and mentally alert. They deeply resent what to them, is a catastrophic attack upon their ability to earn a living and enjoy life."[14]

Treatment of Menopause

Considering that the "disease" had not truly been defined, it is not suprising that the treatments for the condition were often esoteric, to say the least. Leake in 1777 felt that for amenorrhea "It does not appear advisable to use violent means so late in life, with the view to bring back the discharge; but only to carry off the accumulated, superfluous blood, by bleeding and gentle purgatives."[5] "Where the patient is delicate and subject to a female weakness, night sweats or an habitual purging, with flushings in the face and a hectic fever," Leake recommended for treatment "asses milk, jellies, and raw eggs.... At meals she may be indulged with half a pint of old, clear London Porter or a glass of Rhenish wine ... when her strength is increased, and if her lungs and vital parts are sound, she may venture on sea bathing or the cold bath, with great advantage."[5]

Burns, rather wisely, stated that "when the health is good, no particular medicines are requisit; but if there be a tendency to any peculiar disease, then the appropriate remedies must be employed." It is rather a pity that he added as his next, and final instruction, "the bowels must be kept open."[6]

Other forms of therapy had long been described. For example, organotherapy or glandular therapy was a very ancient form of treatment.[15,16] The Egyptians were known to eat the penis of the ass as a cure for impotence. The Greeks and Romans prescribed the testicles of the ass for this purpose.

Such treatments were to become popularized in the late nineteenth century. At the age of 72, Brown-Sequard reported before the Société de Biologie of Paris (June 1, 1888) that he had rejuvenated himself by injections of "testicular juice." The improvement in health manifested itself in greater body vigor, better vesical (sphincteric) action, and better intestinal activity. According to Brown-Sequard, Augusta Brown used testicular extract to combat feminine debility.

At the close of the nineteenth century, ovarian therapy was limited to the administration of crude ovaries, ovarian juice (*suc ovarien*), powdered ovaries, and powdered ovarian tablets. These substances were used for conditions such as physiologic and surgical menopause, dysmenorrhea, and adiposity.[15]

The Development of Estrogenic Hormones

It is generally accepted that the first genuine belief in the existence of an "internal secretion" was voiced by Theophile de Bordeu in 1775. The actual term "internal secretion" was first employed by Claude Bernard in 1855 in a lecture at the Collège de France.[17] Early in this century, William Baylis and E.H. Starling were dissatisfied with the term "internal secretion." They set off in search of a better name and consulted with various people. Included among those whose opinions were valued was William Hardy who, after discussion with W.T. Vesey of Cambridge, suggested the word "hormone."[17]

In 1849 came the first factual discovery of the physiology of the sex organs and their hormones when A.A. Berthold showed that the transplantation of cocks' testes into some other part of the body prevented the atrophy of the coxcomb which usually followed castration. He attributed this result to the influence exerted by the testes on the blood and thence on the body as a whole.[17]

It was not until the present century that the modern conception of ovarian physiology took shape. In 1912 Adler produced the changes of estrus by injecting into virgin animals watery extracts of ovary.[17] Estimation of estrogenic effect on vaginal smears is based on an observation by Stockard and Papanicolaou (1917)[18] that the vaginal epithelium of rodents becomes cornified at the onset of estrus. The reaction occurs not only in mature animals, but also in immature and ovariectomized animals. It was the recognition of this last fact by Allen and Doisy in 1924 that gave origin to their test for the assessment of the activity of estrogens.[19] Estrin was the name given in 1926 by Parkes and Bellerby to the hormone extracted from the ovary by fat solvents.[20]

Butenandt, the Nobel Prize winner mentioned previously, succeeded with other research workers in 1929 in isolating and obtaining in pure form a hormone from the urine of pregnant women which was eventually to be called estrone.[1] Somewhat later estriol was discovered in human pregnancy urine. The structural formula of these hormones was worked out by Butenandt (1930) and others.[21] It was not until 1940 that the presence of B-estradiol was demonstrated in human pregnancy urine and in the placenta. Estradiol is the most effective estrogen in the female that is known today.

A logical development in the history of glandular therapy was the substitution of the newly available estrogens in place of crushed ovaries and the like. As mentioned earlier, this form of treatment became popular from the early 1960s onward, under the general description of estrogen replacement therapy. Initially, reports of this new therapy followed a similar pattern. They generally began with extremely negative statements about the menopause, which were then followed by dramatically positive descriptions for reversal of such effects by the treatment, invariably claiming the properties to be age-preventing. A classic example from this period is the following:

> At the age 50 there are no ova, no follicles, no theca cells, no estrogen — truly a galloping catastrophe. The timely administration of natural estrogens plus an appropriate progestogen to middle-aged women will prevent the climacteric and menopause — a syndrome that seems unnecessary for most of the women in the civilized world. The estrogenic treatment of older women will inhibit osteoporosis and thus help to prevent fractures, as long as they continue healthful activities and appropriate diets. Breasts and genital organs will not shrivel. Such women will be much more pleasant to live with and will not become dull and unattractive.[22]

These reports were not entirely without merit. Some of the observations, although unproven, were astute and based on sound clinical methods. Moreover, the side effect of such publications was to stimulate legitimate in-depth research into the various unsubstantiated claims, with an escalating number of publications in the medical literature.

Surgical Removal of Ovaries

The background to menopause would hardly be complete without a brief consideration of the history of surgical removal of ovaries. In 1685, Justice Theodorus Schorkopff published what appears to be the earliest feature devoted entirely to ovarian cysts.[16] He suggested extirpation as a cure — "provided," he added, "the operation were not too cruel and hazardous." He did not, however, perform the operation, and the contributions of Ephraim McDowell (1771-1830) form the fundamental knowledge upon which abdominal gynecologic surgery rests.

The year 1809 marked an important advance in gynecologic therapy and, indeed, a milestone in abdominal surgery. In that year, McDowell, after 14 years of practice in the frontier town of Danville, Kentucky, successfully performed the first ovariotomy. He fully realized that the procedure was an experimental one and the first report only appeared in 1817.[23] The cyst, which was first emptied of fluid, and then totally excised, weighed 22 pounds. McDowell described this patient's postoperative course as follows: "In five days I visited her, and much to my astonishment found her engaged in making up her bed. I gave her particular caution for the future and in 25 days, she returned home as she came, in good health, which she continues to enjoy."[23]

The medical profession in general failed to give approval to the procedure for many years, and Sir Thomas Spencer Wells (1818-1897) must be "accorded the credit of having placed ovariotomy in the position not only of an acknowledged operation, but one of the most successful of one of the great operations of surgery."[17] Charles Clay (1801-1893) may be called the "father of ovariotomy" in Britain because he performed the first operation in 1842.[17] As time went on he did so many of these operations that he used to reckon his performances by the ton, thinking nothing of referring to 2000 pounds of weight removal of ovarian tumors per month.[17]

Robert Battey (1828-1895) was the first to suggest the operation of oophorectomy for such conditions as dysmenorrhea and neuroses. Battey performed the first oophorectomy on August 27, 1872. He attempted to justify the operation of removal of normal ovaries by stating "The removal of both ovaries puts an end to ovulation entirely and this determines the menopause or change of life; whereby I have hoped, through the intervention of the great nervous revolution which ordinarily accompanies the climacteric, to uproot and remove serious sexual disorders and re-establish the general health." He did qualify this further, perhaps somewhat prophetically, by stating that "I believe these organs should alone be sacrificed for grave causes, and then only as a dernier resort, when the hitherto recognized resources of our art have been expended in vain."[25]

Since the above early development, the operation of bilateral oophorectomy has become a routine practice at hysterectomy performed by some gynecologists. The ostensible reason is to prevent the subsequent development of ovarian malignancy. Heated controversy exists to this day as to the justification for the procedure (see Chapter 10).

CHANGING POPULATION TRENDS

It is difficult to predict the population changes for the future. But it does appear certain that we are going to see an ever increasing number of postmenopausal women. The effect of the so-called population explosion is yet to have its geriatric impact.

The "baby boom" that followed the second world war has had a continuous effect on society. Initially the demand was for infant-care services; later it was for places in schools and colleges. Initially, there were too few maternity hospital beds and schoolteachers; now maternity beds close and teachers go unemployed. The ranks of the baby boom children born between 1946 and 1961 are now moving through young adulthood and will begin to exert a considerable effect when they reach middle age. In other words, after decades of the expanding influence of the youth-oriented culture, a slow but inexorable change is taking place in the population of the developed countries, America in particular, that could change many facets of the way of life.

A second factor to be mentioned at this point is that of birth control. The effect of family limitation, plus the contribution of improved overall health care with increased longevity, are resulting in a gradual aging of the general population. Specifically, the population will continue to increase, probably for decades, but will have a larger proportion of elderly people and a smaller proportion of the young.

It would be presumptuous to attempt to forecast the consequences of this trend. A number of unpredictable factors such as variations in life styles, taste, and new innovations are a few of the difficulties in the way of any guess as to the future. But it does seem unlikely that any aspect of life will be left untouched, including land use, requirements for recreation, fashion trends, medical care, retirement practices, the economy, and politics in general. Much more is bound to be written about this aging of the population, and there is no need to pursue the matter further in this book.

The real meaning of this to the medical profession is of critical importance, and no less to the subject of menopause. In real terms, there are more women who will be spending a greater proportion of their lives in the postmenopausal years. Today, more than half of all Americans are under the age of 30, with about 38 percent between 30 to 64 years, and 11 percent being 65 or older. By the year 2000, the middle-aged will outnumber the young by 46 percent to 42 percent, with 12 percent over 65. A woman at age 50 can expect to live another 30.3 years; 75 years ago she could only have looked forward to another 21.89 years.[25]

Women are still increasing their life expectancy over men: Whereas a 60-year-old white woman's life expectancy was about two years longer than a man's in 1940, it is now five years longer.[25]

Which brings us to the bottom line—the physician is inevitably going to be faced with a "graying" population. Included in this will be more women at the time of menopause with more than one third of their lives ahead of them. And they will have questions and be looking for answers.

References

1.   Butenandt A: Untersuchungen uber das weibliche sexual hormon. Darstellung und eigen schaften des kristallisierten Progynons. Dtsch Med Wochenschr 55: 2171, 1929

2.   Wilson RA: Feminine Forever, New York, Mayflower-Dell, 1966

3.   N Engl J Med. No. 23, Vol. 293, December 4, 1975

4.   Aetios of Amida, translated from Latin edition of Cornarius (1542) by Ricci JV. Philadelphia, Blakiston, 1950

5.   Leake J: Chronic or Slow Diseases Peculiar to Women. London, Baldwin, 1777

6.   Burns J: Diseases of Women and Children. London, Longman, 1814

7.   Charasse H: Advice to a wife. Philadelphia, Lippincott, 1868

8.   Tilt EJ: The change of life in health and disease. London, Churchill, 1857

9.   Colombat de L'Isère M: Treatise on the diseases of females. Translated by Meigs CD, Blanchard L. Philadelphia, Lea, 1845

10.   Borner E: The menopause. In Cyclopaedia of Obstetrics and Gynecology, Vol. II. New York, William Wood, 1887

11.   Wilson RA, Wilson TA: The fate of the nontreated postmenopausal woman. A plea for the maintenance of adequate estrogen from puberty to the grave. J Am Geriatr Soc 11:347, 1963

12.   Wilson RA, Brevetti RE, Wilson TA: Specific procedures for the elimination of the menopause. West J Surg Obstet Gynecol 71:110, 1963

13.   Davis ME: Modern management of menopausal patient. Can Med Dig 33:39, 1966

14.   Rhoades FP: Minimizing the menopause. J Am Geriatr Soc 15:346, 1967

15.   Ricci JV: One hundred years of gynecology, 1800-1900. Philadelphia, Blakiston, 1945

16.   Ricci JV: The genealogy of gynecology 2000 BC-1800 AD, 2nd Ed. Philadelphia, Blakiston, 1950

17.   Kerr JM, Johnstone RW, Phillips MH: Historical Review of British Obstetrics and Gynaecology 1800-1950. London, Livingstone, 1954

18.   Stockard CR, Papanicolaou GN: The existence of a typical oestrus cycle in the guinea pig—with a study of its histological and physiological changes. Am J Anat 22:225, 1917

19.   Allen E, Francis BF, Robertson LL, et al: The hormone of the ovarian follicle: its localization and action in test animals and additional points bearing upon the internal secretions of the ovary. Am J Anat 34:133, 1924

20.   Parkes AS, Bellerby CW: Studies on the internal secretions of the ovary. I The distribution in the ovary of the oestrus-producing hormone. J Physiol 61:562, 1926

21.   Butenandt A: Uber die reindarstellung des follikel-hormons aus schwangerenharn. Z F Physiol Chem 191:127, 1930

22.   Wilson RA, Wilson TA: The basic philosophy of estrogen maintenance. J Am Geriatr Soc 20:521, 1972

23.   McDowell E: Three cases of extirpation of diseased ovaria. Ecleptic Repertory, and Analytical Review, Medical and Philosophical 7:242, 1817

24.   Battey R: Extirpation of the functionally active ovaries for the remedy of otherwise incurable diseases. Trans Am Gynecol Soc 1:101, 1876

25.   US News and World Report: Life expectancy from official reports. Nov. 7, 1977, p 7

2

The Etiology of Menopause

A consideration of the etiology of menopause prompts a question as to whether ovarian failure represents a physiologic or a pathologic event. The search for the answer, which probably lies somewhere between the two, necessitates some knowledge of the pertinent embryology, anatomy, physiology, anthropology, pathology, comparative animal biology, and even a little philosophy.

It is difficult to find a rational explanation for cessation of ovarian function, unless, teleologically speaking, the event be considered a defense mechanism for the species. Thus, women may be expected to cease bearing children at a time of their life when sufficient years remain for the suckling and rearing of their progeny. This is a philosophical area for discussion, with little direct pertinence. The purpose of this chapter will be to review the current available facts.

SPONTANEOUS (NATURAL) MENOPAUSE

Embryogenesis of the Ovary

The development of the gonad, which is first observable in a five- to six-week embryo (7 to 12 mm), commences from three embryonic sources: (1) primordial germ cells; (2) coelomic epithelium; and (3) underlying mesenchyme.

Initially, a swelling is observed on the medial aspect of the *urogenital ridge*, usually called the *gonadal ridge* (Figure 2.1).[1] This results from proliferation of the covering *coelomic epithelium* and the underlying mesenchyme. Finger-like processes gradually extend from the multiplying coelomic epithelial cells into the deeper mesenchyme and are called *primary sex cords*.

The *primordial germ cells* do not arise from the coelomic epithelium. In fact, the coelomic epithelium was previously termed the "germinal epithelium" because of this mistaken idea. The germ cells probably develop from primitive endodermal cells of the wall of the yolk sac.[2] Visible at the fourth week, they migrate, and by the sixth week they reach the developing gonadal mesenchyme and are incorporated in the primary sex cords (Figure 2-2).[1] The gonad, at this stage, is termed an *indifferent gonad*.

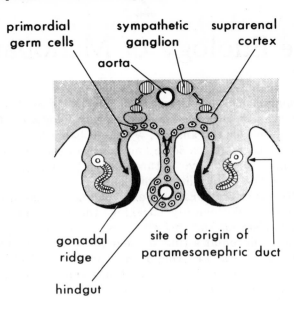

Figure 2-1.   Transverse section of a five-week embryo showing the gonadal ridges and the migration of the primordial germ cells (From Moore KL: The Developing Human, Clinically Oriented Embryology, 2nd ed. Philadelphia, 1977. Courtesy of WB Saunders, Publishers).

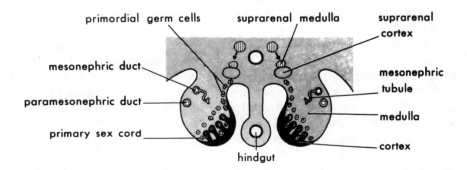

Figure 2-2.   Schematic section of a six-week embryo showing the bipotential indifferent gonads composed of an outer cortex and inner medulla (From Moore KL: The Developing Human, Clinically Oriented Embryology, 2nd ed. Philadelphia, 1977. Courtesy of WB Saunders, Publishers).

Further gonadal differentiation depends upon the sex chromosome makeup of the individual. The presence of a Y chromosome induces testis formation, and its absence will allow for the formation of an ovary.[1] For a while, irrespective of the future path, the sex cords develop and the primordial germ cells are progressively embedded. In the testes, they will eventually differentiate into the seminiferous tubules, but, if the gonad is to be an ovary, these primordial cell cords will break up into clusters and gradually differentiate into *primordial ovarian follicles* (Figure 2-3).[3]

The primordial ovarian follicles actually develop slowly and the ovary, as such, can only be identified properly by about the tenth or eleventh week of embryonic life. The breaking up of the sex cords into primordial follicles starts at about the sixteenth week. Each primordial follicle is made up of a primordial germ cell, now called an *oogonium,* which is encircled by a single layer of *follicular cells* derived from the cortical sex cords.[1,3]

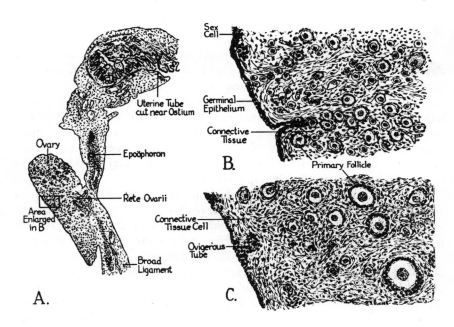

Figure 2-3.   Ovary toward the close of intrauterine life. (A) Projection drawing, X10, of ovary, uterine tube, and broad ligament of an eight-month fetus. (B) Projection drawing, X150, of part of ovary indicated by rectangle in A. (C) Projection drawing, X150, of a similarly located section from ovary of a newborn infant (From Patten BM: Human Embryology. New York, 1968. Courtesy of McGraw-Hill, Publishers).

A major unexplained difference between testis and ovary is the ability of the former to produce new spermatagonia into old age, and the inability of the ovary to ever produce new eggs after birth. In fact, many thousands of oogonia develop by active mitosis of primitive germ cells during fetal life and some two million will become primary oocytes by the time of birth. No further oogonia will ever be produced after birth.[1]

The follicles are surrounded by the remains of the primitive mesenchyme, which is now called the *ovarian stroma.* The coelomic (germinal) epithelium covering the ovary thins out to a single layer by the time of birth. It is separated from the follicles by a thin fibrous capsule called the *tunica albuginea.*[1] The ovary, therefore, is the only intraperitoneal organ not covered by true peritoneum.

The fully developed ovary will thus consist essentially of two major components: (1) primordial follicles, and (2) stromal tissue.

Aging of the Ovary

The ovary, with its complement of follicles, will tend to remain quiescent until puberty. The details of puberty, menarche, and the reproductive age are not the subject of this book.

Throughout the reproductive years there is a progressive loss of follicles as a continuous process. Nonetheless, there is ample evidence that oocytes may still be found in the ovary after the cessation of menstruation.[4-8] It is possible that these few remaining oocytes are abnormal,[9] although ultrastructural studies suggest the follicle and its oocyte to usually be quite normal in appearance.[10]

Information on the actual numbers of oocytes in relation to age is sparse. The best quantitative counts of oocytes in the human ovary are those of Bloch,[5,6] from whom the numbers in Table 2.1 are worth considering. The range is seen to be extremely wide. But there is a progressive decline in the number of follicles with age.

Following menopause, the ovary becomes smaller, slightly fibrotic, and the surface is pitted. Ultrastructural studies show extremely interesting changes. Whereas the diminution of primordial follicles with the increase in fibroblasts and connective tissue is confirmed, the stromal (interstitial) cells apparently become more abundant.[10] The morphologic result is an atrophy of the ovarian cortex which once housed most of the oocytes, and an apparent hyperplasia of the medulla where most of the interstitial cells are found.

The ovarian structural changes directly parallel the endocrine changes, to be outlined in the next chapter. Theca interna and granulosa cells, the usual sources of estrogen and progesterone, are gradually lost, whereas the stromal (interstitial) cells become more abundant and active. The stromal cells are a probable source of androgens.[11,12]

Table 2-1. The Relationship Between Age and the Number of Oocytes Present in the Human Ovary

Number of Females	Age Years	Number of Primordial Follicles	Range
5	6–9	484,000	258,000–755,000
5	12–16	382,000	85,000–591,000
7	18–24	155,000	39,000–290,000
11	25–31	59,000	8,100–228,000
8	32–38	74,000	15,000–208,000
7	40–44	8,300	350–28,000

Adapted from Bloch: Acta Anat 14:108, 1952

Reproductive Aging in Laboratory Animals

Climacteric was long considered to be an event unique to the human female. Animals, it was thought, did not lose their reproductive capacity, as did women. This is not true. The reason for the ignorance concerning reproductive aging in animals lies, of course, in the animal's natural history. They live in a world of survival of the fittest, and age in the animal world usually leads to "accidental death." Nor, until the last decade or so, were many animals allowed to age under observation in research laboratories. One colony that did allow such natural aging was that of van Wagenen,[13] who established a unique monkey colony in 1935 and studied the animals for the next forty years. Even now, information is limited, but there have been findings of considerable interest.[13-15] In particular, van Wagenen has been able to report on the complete life cycle including menstrual and reproductive histories of three monkeys whose dates of birth are accurately known.[13]

Most animals show a reduced litter size with age, and the actual production of fetuses usually ceases well before death. But few animals have been shown to lose their reproductive capacity by virtue of the aging process of the ovary described above. The mechanism of the reduction of fertility in most animals appears to lie outside of the ovary, and there is considerable evidence for continued cyclic ovarian activity in most species until death or very close to it.[14,15] Nonetheless, the animals do manifest a reduction in reproductive capacity by gradual decline in number of fetuses per litter. The reason for the decrease in litter size is outside the scope of this book, but it may relate to a decline in the ability of the blastocyst to make a satisfactory union with the aging uterus.[15] This could, in turn, be due to autoimmune factors, hormonal changes, and even alterations caused by aging within DNA itself.

Quantitative estimates of total numbers of oocytes throughout the lifespan are known for some animals.[6] Not surprisingly, follicles are present in most species until death. This accounts for the above finding in captive animals that, although fertility ceases, the reproductive cycle continues for a species-specific time, probably genetically determined, and usually extending virtually until death.[14]

However, in some animals, the ovaries do apparently as in the human female, become oocyte depleted. In mice, for example, the rate at which oocytes are lost differs between strains. Thus, in most strains, a complement of around 100 primordial follicles remains at 800 days. But there is one strain called the CBA type which shows no residual oocytes at 450 days.[16] Information about other animals, except the rhesus monkey,[13,17] is relatively limited. The reproductive cycle activity in different species, expressed as a percentage of the total lifespan, is summarized in

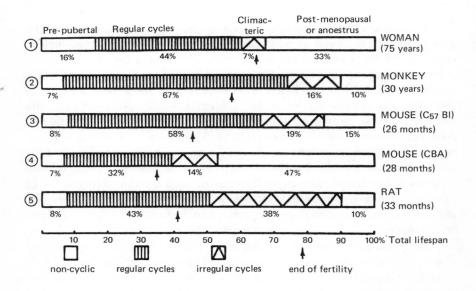

Figure 2–4.   Reproductive cyclic activity expressed as a percentage of total lifespan. The end of the reproductive phase of the monkey is an estimate based on three observations by van Wagenen.[13] (From Hones: In van Keep, Lauritzen (eds): Front Hormone Res 3:5, 1975. Courtesy of S. Karger, Publishers).

Figure 2.4. It is striking that women and the CBA strain of mouse appear to be fairly unique in having a long noncyclic phase.

The lack of an animal model for the study of the pathophysiology of human menopause has long hindered research. It would appear as if the CBA strain of mouse and the rhesus monkey could provide such a model.[13,4,17] Patterns of vaginal bleeding and serum hormone profiles consistent with those described in peri- and postmenopause have been described in the rhesus monkey.[17] If such a model can be used to objectively test the endocrine and metabolic outcome of manipulating the steroid hormone milieu, then the hope of acquiring meaningful answers to important questions about the cause and effect of reproductive aging should lie in the not too distant future.

Age of Menopause

There is considerable evidence that the age at which the onset of menstruation (menarche) occurs is falling.[18] For example, the age of menarche reported as 15.5 years in Britain in 1855, had fallen to 13.1 years a century later.[19,20] This appears to be a well-substantiated finding, and although attributed to improved health, nutrition, and general socioeconomic conditions, is really unexplained. This falling age of menarche has long led to the assumption that the average age of menopause might be rising. The probability is that this is not so.

The many observations made as to the age of onset of menopause in medieval Europe cannot be written off as absurdities. These findings have been reviewed by Amundsen and Diers,[21] from whom Table 2.2 has been derived. It is striking that the majority of medieval sources reported menopause to occur at an average age of 50 years.

Recent studies have tended to confirm the menopause to be occurring at about the same age. Frommer found the modal and median age of menopause to be 50.1 years, using a method of study called the probit transformation.[22] This is a method allowing the proportion of women at any particular age who have reached their menopause to be calculated without knowing the age of menopause of any of the women being surveyed. All that is required are the following two pieces of information about any woman: (1) whether she has reached menopause; and (2) her current age when providing the information. Provided that sufficient women are used in the investigation, the percentage of women at any age who have reached the menopause can be calculated with a high degree of accuracy.[23] Using similar study models, McKinlay et al. reported the median age of menopause to be 50.78 years.[24] Another probit analysis, this time of South African black women, reported the median age for menopause to be 50.70 years.[25]

Table 2-2.   Average Age of Menopause According to Some Medieval
Sources

Author	Century	Average Age Cited
Aetius	6th	50
Paulus Aegineta	7th	50
"Trotula"	11th/12th	50
Hildegard	12th	50
Thomas of Cantimpre	13th	50
Gilbertus Anglicus	13th	50
John of Gaddesden	14th	50
Ortolff the Bavarian	15th	40–50

Adapted from Amundsen and Diers: Hum Biol 45:605, 1973

The general consensus appears to be that natural menopause will occur in industrialized societies at a median age of about 50. There is, therefore, no evidence that this median age has tended to increase. Nor does there appear to be any indication of a relation between the age of menarche and menopause. Moreover, age of menopause does not appear to depend on socioeconomic conditions, race, marital status, income, geography, parity, height, or skinfold thickness.[26]

Do any factors influence the age of menopause? One possibility does exist, and that is cigarette smoking. There are indications that smokers, as a group, have an earlier natural menopause than do nonsmokers.[27,27A] This relationship was found to exist in two large independent sets of data analyzed by the Boston Collaborative Drug Surveillance Program, and was similar both in the United States and other countries. Furthermore, heavier smokers were more likely to be postmenopausal, for any given age, than light smokers. Having smoked and stopped increased the chance of being menopausal, as compared to a woman who had never smoked, although there was a decreased possibility when compared to a current smoker.[27,27A] The mechanism is unexplained, but it is theorized that the metabolism of steroid hormones may be influenced by certain liver-metabolizing enzymes[28] which are induced by the content of cigarette smoke.[29] Another theory involves the direct actions of nicotine on the neuroendocrine system.[30]

Premature Ovarian Failure and Antiovarian Antibodies

Premature ovarian failure is essentially unexplained. It has been theorized that the condition may be due to the development of antibodies either to ovarian tissue[31] or to FSH.[32] Autoantibodies to cytoplasmic components of the ovary have been reported in patients with premature ovarian failure[33,33A] and other proven disorders.[34] For example, patients with autoimmune Addison's disease have a high incidence of premature ovarian failure associated with IgG antibodies in their serum, reactive with the adrenal cortex, and also to steroid-producing cells in the ovary.[34] Conversely, patients with tuberculous Addison's disease do not.

Urinary FSH derived from patients with premature ovarian failure does seem to be biologically active.[35] Furthermore, these patients will not respond to exogenous, biologically active FSH, even when the ovaries are known to contain numerous primordial follicles.[36] It is of course possible that failure to respond or to ovulate could be due to anti-FSH antibodies,[33] but much work is still necessary before the exact nature of the abnormality can be elucidated.

ARTIFICIAL MENOPAUSE

Radiation Menopause

The use of radiation for induction of menopause, usually in cases of dysfunctional uterine bleeding, has been largely superseded by hysterectomy. Nonetheless, it is still employed in some centers and for this reason is worthy of discussion.

There are two described techniques for induction of menopause with radiation:

1. The first involves the exposure of both ovaries to 300 to 600 of deep x-rays, usually given in divided doses.
2. The second method is the insertion of 50 mg of radium into the cavity of the uterus for 40 hours. Doses in excess of 2500 mg hours cause extensive endometrial necrosis and cervical stenosis.

Radiation menopause has the advantages of inducing amenorrhea with avoidance of surgical risks in poor operative candidates. The treatment, moreover, has virtually no immediate risk, provided the recommended doses are not exceeded.[37]

There are, however, many potential disadvantages:

1. Cancer risk: It is possible that patients treated by radiation have an increased liability to the development of malignant disease in the genital tract.[38] There are controversial views and it is difficult to

know whether subsequent development of the genital tract malignancy is a direct sequel to the radiotherapy itself, or merely an indication that perimenopausal bleeding constitutes a high-risk group
for genital malignancy. Thus, Bamford and Wagman reported 6
malignant tumors of the genital tract out of 93 patients undergoing
radiation menopause,[38] whereas Turnbull, in another series, could
find no evidence that women treated by radium were more likely
than average to develop cancer of the body of the uterus.[39] He even
suggested that in his series the mortality from subsequent development of uterine cancer was possibly balanced by the high mortality
of hysterectomy as compared to radiotherapy.[39] One definite com-
ment can be made. Radiation, unlike hysterectomy, cannot reduce
the likelihood of uterine cancer, and with operative mortality rates
now so low, hysterectomy should supersede radiation in all but the
poor risk patients.

2. Radiation burns: The two methods described above can both result
    in systemic effects (radiation sickness). Moreover radiation burns of
    the bladder and rectum are possible.
3. Fetal malformation: Women aged 40 or less may not be permanently
    sterilized by this method. Ovulatory function can recur, and obvi-
    ously conception could even precede menstruation. The theoretical
    risk of genetic abnormality and fetal malformation thus exists.[37]
4. Menopausal symptoms: Radiation menopause may be followed by
    severe menopausal symptoms. Hot flushes, loss of libido, and necro-
    tic changes leading to vaginal discharge and dyspareunia are the
    most frequent of these unpleasant symptoms, which can occur in up
    to 47 percent of cases.[40]

The current consensus favors hysterectomy, and radiation menopause is only rarely indicated. If a patient receives such therapy or has
in her previous history, then she should be seen annually for a full
gynecologic checkup, including cytological examination. She must also
be instructed to report any episode of vaginal bleeding.

Surgical Menopause

Menopause will follow in the women of reproductive age if the
ovaries are surgically removed. The operation of bilateral oophorectomy
(ovariectomy, castration) is not usually done alone, but most frequently
accompanies removal of the uterus.

The surgical removal of normal ovaries at the time of routine abdominal hysterectomy performed for benign conditions is a controversial subject in modern gynecology. The arguments for and against
removing ovaries are listed below.

The reasons usually advanced for removal of ovaries are as follows:

1. Prevention of subsequent development of cancer in the retained ovaries.
2. The theory that retained ovaries have diminished or absent function.
3. High incidence of repeat laparotomy for ovarian pathology.

These ovaries are frequently retained in order to:

1. Prevent development of postoperative menopausal symptoms (Chapter 7).
2. Prevent regressive effects related to estrogen withdrawal (Chapter 4).
3. Prevent development of osteoporosis (Chapter 5).
4. Prevent development of coronary heart disease (Chapter 6).
5. Prevent potential adverse psychological reactions.

The above mentioned factors will be dealt with in depth in Chapter 10, where current opinion is evaluated and specific guidelines given as to the handling of ovaries during surgery. Prior to that it is important to understand the essential basic principles described in the next five chapters.

References

1. Moore KL: The Developing Human—Clinically Oriented Embryology. Philadelphia, Saunders, 1977

2. Witschi E: Migration of the germ cells of human embryos from the yolk sac to the primitive gonadal folds. Contrib Embryol Carnegie Inst 32:67, 1948

3. Patten BM: Human Embryology. New York, McGraw-Hill, 1968

4. Mandl AM, Zuckerman S: The relation of age to numbers of oocytes. J Endocrinol 7:190, 1951

5. Bloch E: Quantitative morphological investigations of the follicular system in women. Variations at different ages. Acta Anat 14:108, 1952

6. Bloch E: A quantitative morphological investigation of the follicular system in newborn female infants. Acta Anat 17:201, 1953

7. Mandl AM, Shelton M: A quantitative study of oocytes in young and old nulliparous rats. J Endocrinol 18:444, 1959

8. Jones EC, Krohn PL: The relationship between age, numbers of oocytes and fertility in virgin and multiparous mice. J Endocrinol 21:469, 1961

9. Hertig AT: The aging ovary. J Clin Endocrinol Metab 4:581, 1944

10.   Costoff A: An ultrastructural study of ovarian changes in the menopause. In Greenblatt RB, Mahesh UB, McDonough PG, eds: The Menopausal Syndrome. New York, Medcom, 1974, p 12

11.   Smith OW, Ryan KJ: Estrogen in the human ovary. Am J Obstet Gynecol 84:141, 1962

12.   Rice BF, Savard K: Steroid hormone formation in the ovary. J Clin Endocrinol 26:593, 1966

13.   van Wagen G: Vital statistics from a breeding colony. J Med Primatol 1:3, 1972

14.   Jones EC: The post-reproductive phase in mammals. In Estrogens in the Postmenopause. Front Hor Res 3:1, Basel, Karger, 1975

15.   Finn CA: Investigations into reproductive aging in experimental animals. In Beard RD (ed): The Menopause. Lancaster, MTP Press, 1976

16.   Jones EC, Krohn PL: The relationship between age, numbers of oocytes and fertility in virgin and multiparous mice. J Endocrinol 21:469, 1961

17.   Hodgen GD, Goodman AL, O'Connor A, Johnson DK: Menopause in rhesus monkeys. Model for study of disorders in the human climacteric. Am J Obstet Gynecol 127:581, 1977

18.   Tanner JM: Growth at Adolescence, 2nd ed. Oxford, Blackwell, 1962

19.   Brand PC: Age at Menopause. Elve/Labor Vincit, Leiden, 1978

20.   Wilson DC, Sutherland I: The present age of the menarche in Southern England. J Obstet Gynaecol Br Emp 67:320, 1960

21.   Amundsen DW, Diers CJ: The age of menopause in medieval Europe. Hum Biol 45:605, 1973

22.   Frommer DJ: Changing age of menopause. Br Med J 2:349, 1964

23.   Finney DJ: Probit Analysis, 2nd ed. London, Cambridge University Press, 1952

24.   McKinlay S, Jefferys M, Thompson B: An investigation of the age at menopause. J Biosoc Sci 4:161, 1972

25.   Frere G: Mean age at menopause and menarche in South Africa. S Afr J Med Sci 36:21, 1971

26.   MacMahon B, Worcester J: Age at menopause. National Center for Health Statistics, series 11, no. 19, Washington, DC, 1966

27.   Jick H, Porter J, Morrison AS: Relation between smoking and age of natural menopause. Lancet i:1354, 1977

27A.   Linquist O, Bengtsson C: The effect of smoking on menopausal age. Maturitas 1:171, 1979

28.   Conney AH, Jacobson M, Schneidman K, Kuntzman R: Induction of liver microsomal cortisol 6B-hydroxylase by diphenylhydantoin of phenobarbital. Life Sci 4:1091, 1965

29.   Beckett AH, Triggs EJ: Enzyme induction in man caused by smoking. Nature 216:587, 1967

30.   Goodman LS, Gilman A: The Pharmacological Basis of Therapeutics. New York, MacMillan, 1975, p 568

31.   Vallotton MB, Forbes AP: Antibodies to cytoplasm of ova. Lancet 2:264, 1966

32.   Starup J, Sele V, Henriksen B: Amenorrhea associated with increased production of gonadothrophins and morphologically normal ovarian follicular apparatus. Acta Endocrinol 66:248, 1971

33.   deMoraes-Ruehsen M, Blizzard RM, Garcia-Bunuel R, Jones GS: Autoimmunity and ovarian failure. Am J Obstet Gynecol 112:693, 1972

33A.   Coulam CB, Ryan RJ: Premature Menopause I. Etiology. Am J Obstet Gynecol 133:639, 1979

34.   Irvine WJ; Autoimmune mechanisms in endocrine disease. Proc R Soc Med 67:499, 1974

35.   Jones GS, deMoraes-Ruehsen M: A new syndrome of amenorrhea in association with hypergonadotropism and apparently normal ovarian follicular apparatus. Am J Obstet Gynecol 104:597, 1969

36.   Duignan NM, Shaw RS, Glass MR, Butt WR, Edwards RH: Sex hormone levels and gonadotrophin release in premature ovarian failure. Br J Obstet Gynaecol 85:862, 1978

37.   Jeffcoate N: Principles of Gynaecology, 4th ed. London, Butterworths, 1975, p 532

38.   Bamford DS, Wagman H: Radium menopause: a long-term follow-up. J Obstet Gynaecol Br Cwlth 79:82, 1972

39.   Turnbull AC: Radiation menopause or hysterectomy. J Obstet Gynaecol Br Emp 63:179, 1956

40.   McLaren HC: Effects of the radium menopause. Br Med J 2:76, 1950

3
Endocrinology of Climacteric

There is one popular fallacy that needs exposure at the outset: The endocrine difference between a premenopausal and a postmenopausal woman is not simply a matter of estrogen deficiency. There are numerous subtle changes that commence almost a decade before menopause and continue for many years after. The purpose of this chapter is to outline these changes.

GENERAL PRINCIPLES

This short manual does not claim to be a textbook of endocrinology. Nonetheless, some brief general principles of female endocrinology will be helpful to the clinician in understanding the specific hormonal events that take place around menopause.

The Hormones

A hormone is a chemical messenger, produced by specialized glandular tissue, that is released into the blood stream, and which is able to initiate specific effects on distant responsive cells. The three groups of hormones of importance to the female in relation to reproductive function and menopause are:

1. *Releasing factors* from the hypothalamus: gonadotropin releasing hormone (GnRH), also called luteinizing hormone releasing factor (LHRF), and follicle stimulating hormone releasing factor (FSHRF). There is still debate whether the luteinizing hormone and follicle stimulating hormone releasing factor are the same substance. For the purpose of this monograph, they will be referred to collectively as GnRH.
2. *Pituitary gonadotropins (follicle stimulating hormone* [FSH] and *luteinizing hormone* [LH] from the anterior pituitary).
3. *Sex steroids (estrogens, progesterone, androgens)* from the ovary and adrenal glands and from extraglandular metabolism.

These hormones essentially induce responses in tissues possessing specific cellular receptors that are able to bind the hormone. The mechanisms vary. A steroid hormone, for example, is bound by a receptor within the cellular cytoplasm and transports it to the nucleus where the hormone will give a specific message to the nuclear chromatin. The latter will respond in a manner that is specific and characteristic. Simplistically, these responses are as follows:

1. GnRH induces the pituitary gland to release FSH and LH.
2. FSH stimulates maturation of the primordial ovarian follicle with resultant steroidogenesis by follicular cells. In particular, FSH will induce synthesis of estradiol. LH is also required in this follicular phase.
3. LH stimulates egg release and formation of the corpus luteum. The steriodogenic effect of the corpus luteum is the synthesis of progesterone in addition to estradiol.
4. Immediately following ovarian steroidogenesis, the specific steroids are released into the blood stream and transported throughout the body. As mentioned above, individual steroids will be selectively bound by tissue cells with specific receptors. For example, estradiol will be bound in vaginal epithelial cells and will induce epithelial growth and maturation.[1]

Serum Levels

Hormones are released into the veins of the specific organs in which they are produced and thence into the general circulation. Blood levels will therefore vary, depending upon the point of collection. The synthesis and release of hormone will also vary from moment to moment and from day to day. This cyclicity creates difficulties in interpretation of single samples and necessitates, in many instances, the collection of serial samples.[2,3]

Although the hormones are probably homogenously distributed in the circulation, they do not all circulate in the same manner. Over 40 percent of estradiol and testosterone, for example, circulate bound to a beta globulin protein carrier called either *estrogen binding globulin* (EBG), *testosterone binding globulin* (TBG), or collectively, *sex hormone binding globulin* (SHBG). A further 58 percent, more or less, is bound to albumin which leaves less than 2 percent to circulate in the free or unbound state. The regular clinical assays usually measure the total circulating hormone unless specific procedures are undertaken to separate the bound from the free level.[4]

Separation of bound hormone from free circulating levels has clinical relevance. The active hormonal properties exist in the free hormone whereas the bound hormone appears to be physiologically inactive.[1]

These hormones are measured in plasma by radioligand competitive protein binding methods, which include radioimmunoassay. The precise data that has been accumulated by these methods has allowed the ovarian and pituitary cycles of the reproductive hormones to be fully defined.[1,4]

Hormone Secretion Rate and Production Rate

Steroid hormone concentrations in ovarian vein and peripheral vein blood have been measured and compared in pre- and postmenopausal subjects. As a result it has been possible to determine which ovarian structures act as a source of the various hormones. Such studies have also provided direct evidence of the rates of hormonal secretion, i.e., it is possible to measure direct glandular secretion.

The *secretion rate* of a hormone will only be equal to the *production rate* if there is no other source for the hormone. That is, a plasma level of a hormone may be made up of various components. Part will be in circulation as a result of direct glandular secretion, the rate of which can be measured. Part may be in circulation following conversion at an extraglandular site of a precursor which has been secreted elsewhere.[5,6] In the postmenopausal woman, estrogen can be derived from androgen.[6,7]

It is possible to define these proportions by use of radioisotopic tracer studies, a subject beyond the scope of this book.[5] In summary, however:

Secretion rate = specific synthesis and release from the endocrine gland.

Production rate = secretion rate + contribution of peripheral conversion of precursors.

Metabolic Clearance Rate

The hormones produced are gradually eliminated from the body. The concept of "clearance" is identical to that of renal clearance. Thus, the *metabolic clearance rate* (MCR) is the rate at which the hormone is irrevocably cleared by organs and tissues of the whole body. In other terms, it is the amount or volume of blood cleared of the hormone in a specific period of time. Once the MCR has been measured, the blood production rate is easily calculated. It is the MCR multiplied by the circulating concentration of that specific hormone.[8]

Receptor Activity and Tissue Effects

From the preceding discussion it becomes apparent, in theory at least, that hormonal activity in an individual can be measured in several ways. These include measurement of specific hormone levels and their metabolites in peripheral venous blood, venous blood from the gland itself, or in 24-hour urine collections, or by the study of secretion rates, production rates, and metabolic clearance rates.

Bioassay is another way to determine hormonal activity. This is dependent upon the uptake of the hormone by the tissue receptors, and then measuring the specific tissue response that occurs. This type of test was of course described long before it was possible to actually measure hormones directly. A specific example of this approach is the evaluation of the cellular pattern of the vaginal smear, a subject which will be dealt with in detail in Chapter 4. Another example is the hormonal effect on endometrium, also an important subject to be discussed in Chapter 4. Such responses are usually called "target tissue" effects.

The so-called "target tissues" can be characterized by the presence of highly specific protein receptor molecules within the cells which bind firmly to the specific circulating steroid.[9-11] Receptors are being demonstrated in many tissues such as ovary, endometrium, hypothalamus, and vaginal epithelium. The absence of a specific hormone receptor in a tissue would result in that tissue being unresponsive to the relevant hormone.

The total number of available binding sites does seem to vary. For example, there are probably more such sites present in tissues under constant estrogen stimulus than would be the case after menopause. Administration of estrogen after menopause results in a gradual increase in binding sites to a premenopausal amount. The delay in tissue response to hormone therapy could be accounted for by this fact.[9]

The reaction between the hormone and the protein receptor molecule, and its subsequent transfer into the nucleus, appear to be similar for all target tissues. But the actual cellular response will depend upon the character of the cell nucleus and will, therefore, vary from one tissue to another.[9] The nature of these tissue responses will be discussed in the next chapter.

The actual cellular mechanism of action of specific hormones is a subject of intense current interest. Simplistically, the tropic hormones act at the level of the cell membranes, a reaction involving adenylate cyclase. The steroid hormones, as alluded to previously, diffuse across the cell membrane into the cellular cytoplasm where they bind to specific protein receptor molecules. The specificity of the protein receptor molecule is remarkably high. The receptor bound steroid then crosses the nuclear chromatin, that is, to the DNA-RNA-protein-lipid complex that represents the genetic apparatus of the resting cell. The steroid receptor complex thus influences which genes are activated by being transcribed into RNA.

Summary

The pertinence of the above information is as follows: The ovary is an extremely important structure, capable during a woman's reproductive age of producing eggs and sex hormones (sex steroids). There is a close interrelationship on a push-pull basis between this activity and the hypothalamic-pituitary hormone-secreting complex.

The ovarian reproductive cycle each month is a repetitive self-cycling mechanism which will continue as long as the ovary is capable of response, that is, for as long as there are primordial ovarian follicles present. Once the ovary becomes follicle depleted, the entire reproductive cycle, with hormone synthesis and release, will fail. This will be reflected in a change of hormonal secretion patterns, production rates, receptor effect, and metabolic clearance.

It must be emphasized that the ovary is not the only source of sex steroids in the human female. The adrenal glands also produce these hormones, albeit in far lesser amounts. Moreover, the adrenal gland and the ovary are able to provide steroid precursors which can be peripherally metabolized to more potent sex hormones. This activity, too, will change after the menopause. It is all these changes that will now be considered in depth.

SEX STEROID HORMONES

Premenopausal

During the reproductive years, the main source of *estradiol* (E_2) is direct secretion by the ovaries. The estradiol is produced cyclically and the ovary accounts for over 90 percent of the total body production. There are several good reports documenting this cyclic production.[1,12] Specifically, there is a gradual increase in production through the cycle to a late follicular peak, prior to ovulation. There is then a fall, followed by a second peak, termed the *luteal maximum,* and then a progressive decrease in value until the start of the next cycle. It is important to note that almost all the estradiol is a result of glandular secretion.

Estrone (E_1), unlike estradiol, is almost equally produced by glandular secretion and by peripheral conversion of androstenedione, testosterone, and estradiol.

The *androstenedione* is produced by both the ovaries and the adrenals, with the adrenal probably being the major producer of the two glands.

Testosterone arises from peripheral conversion of androstenedione to even a larger extent than does estrone. Thus testosterone production is made up of ovarian and adrenal components amounting to 40 percent, and peripheral conversion accounting for the remaining 60 percent. Androgen production also tends to show a cyclic activity although to a lesser extent than estrogen.[13]

The cyclic activity of the ovary and the episodic nature of adrenal hormone secretion make any relative assessment of ovarian and adrenal androgen contribution very difficult. The ovary may, in fact, be a more important source than the adrenal.[14,15]

A most important concept to understand is that the total sex-steroid hormone production in the premenopausal female is made up of two components. There is a relatively constant basal level of estrogen, principally estrone produced by peripheral conversion (extraglandular formation) from androstenedione. On this is superimposed the second component, namely, a fluctuating secretion of estradiol from the developing graafian follicles and corpus luteum. There is also a constant production of androgens with a small proportion contributed by cyclic activity.

Perimenopausal

With the approach of menopause the menstrual cycle becomes irregular and clinical data suggest that the climacteric, or transistional phase of the reproductive period, begins as much as eight years before menopause.[16] Much information is still necessary to clarify the pituitary-ovarian relationship during this waning period of reproductive life.

There have been several comparative studies of the circulating concentrations of gonadotropins, prolactin, and sex steroids of women of different ages before and after the menopause.[17-21] Ovarian estrogen production does not appear to alter before menopause, and ovulation continues, although luteal levels of progesterone appear to decline.[17] However, there is not universal agreement[19,22] in this area and further studies appear to be necessary before excluding the possibility that a slight decrement in estradiol production may explain the gonadotropin rise in premenopausal women.[17,23]

It is not yet clear whether in perimenopausal women the ovaries are under maximum stimulation by the pituitary or whether they are still capable of responding to stimulation with gonadotropic hormones.[24,25] A significant change does, in fact, occur in the hypothalamic-pituitary mechanism before menopause, and this will be discussed later in this chapter.

Postmenopausal

The postmenopause is not a sudden time of estrogen quiescence. Certainly, following menopause, estradiol no longer manifests its cyclic changes and its contribution to total circulating estrogen becomes substantially reduced. The production of estrone, however, is not dramatically reduced. In fact, in postmenopausal women estrogen production is principally, if not completely, the result of peripheral aromatization of plasma androstenedione and not ovarian or adrenal secretion.[7,13,26] Moreover, the amount of androstenedione production and peripheral conversion can vary considerably under different circumstances, including obesity and aging.[27]

PLASMA LEVELS   The loss of cyclicity of estradiol secretion becomes apparent very early. Otherwise, plasma levels tend to remain fairly stable. The average plasma concentrations of the sex steroids are shown on Table 3-1, comprehensively derived from several references.[28-32] The compilation of such a table is open to numerous sources of error, but it does serve to highlight the following features:

1. Premenopausally, the development and regression of the graafian follicle and corpus luteum is reflected in predictable fluctuation of the plasma sex steroid levels.
2. Following spontaneous menopause the levels of estradiol and estrone drop but, as expected, the estrone to a relatively lesser extent than the estradiol. In fact, the amount of precursor androstenedione also drops but the rate of conversion to estrone increases. The result is a relatively stable production of estrone for many years after the menopause.
3. Oophorectomy after menopause appears to have little influence on estradiol and estrone levels whereas an affect similar to spontaneous menopause occurs following oophorectomy in a woman of reproductive age. The extent of the ovarian contribution to plasma estradiol levels is demonstrated by the rapidity with which these levels fall after premenopausal oophorectomy. Significant differences can be demonstrated as early as the first postoperative day.[32]
4. In normal cycling women there is a small but significant cyclicity of plasma androstenedione and testosterone levels. It is possible that stress may increase adrenal production of androstenedione.
5. Removal of ovaries in both pre- and postmenopausal women results in significant reduction of testosterone and androstenedione levels. It would appear that the postmenopausal ovary could be responsible for as much as 50 percent of plasma testosterone and 30 percent of androstenedione levels.[33]
6. Progesterone production is essentially a function of the corpus luteum.

PRODUCTION AND METABOLIC CLEARANCE RATES   There is a decrease in the metabolic clearance rates (MCR) of estrogens and androgens after the menopause.[28,31] The calculated blood production rates are also lower in postmenopausal women than for

Table 3–1. Serum Sex Steroid Concentrations in pg/ml Before and After Spontaneous Menopause and Oophorectomy

	Estrone (E₁)	Estradiol (E₂)	Estriol (E₃)	Progesterone	Testosterone	Androstenedione
Premenopausal women						
Early follicular	25–50	25–75	7–8	100–500	200–400	1600–1750
Late follicular	150–200	200–600			300–800	1850–2000
Mid luteal	70–100	100–300	10–12		300–600	
Oophorectomy before menopause	20–40	15–25		50	75–150	600–1500
Postmenopausal women						
Spontaneous	20–40	9–15	6	100–200	200–300	600–900
Oophorectomy after menopause	20–40	9–15		100–200	100–150	500–800

Data derived from references 28–32.

any other time of the cycle in the premenopausal female. However, the production rates of estrone are not as reduced as are those for estradiol. The reason for this is the previously referred to peripheral conversion of androstenedione to estrone. The metabolic clearance rates for these steroid hormones are as follows:[7,30]

Estrone (E_1) — The MCR of about 2210 ± 120 (MCR liters/24 hour $\pm$ Standard Error) before the menopause declines to 1610 ± 110 after menopause.

Estradiol (E_2) — The premenopausal MCR of about 1350 ± 40 (L/24h $\pm$ SE) drops to 910 ± 70 liters per day after the menopause.

Androstenedione — The premenopausal MCR of about 2000 liters per day decreases to 1850 after menopause.

Testosterone — The premenopausal MCR of about 800 ± 50 liters per day drops to approximately 400 ± 50.

SOURCES OF PRODUCTION

It is pertinent at this time to summarize the sources of production of the sex steroids. These are as follows:

1. Estrone (E_1)
   a. Premenopause
      1. Direct ovarian secretion.
      2. Extraglandular conversion of androstenedione, testosterone, and estradiol.
   b. Postmenopause
      1. Almost totally from peripheral conversion of androstenedione. The actual size of the peripheral conversion of androstenedione may be in adipose tissue.[7]
2. Estradiol (E_2)
   a. Premenopause
      1. Almost totally by direct ovarian secretion.
      2. Small contribution from extraglandular conversion of estrone, androstenedione, and testosterone.
      3. Minimal adrenal contribution possible.
   b. Postmenopause
      1. Extraglandular formation from estrone, androstenedione, and testosterone.
      2. Very little direct ovarian secretion.
3. Androstenedione
      1. Almost no peripheral conversion exists. Virtually all derived from direct glandular secretion.[30,34,35] In postmenopause about 30 percent is contributed by ovary and the rest by the adrenal.[33]

4. Testosterone
   1. Direct secretion from the postmenopausal ovary can account for up to 50 percent.[33] Testosterone levels fall about half in premenopausal patients after oophorectomy.[30]
   2. The adrenal can directly secrete testosterone, but is a lesser source.[15]
   3. Peripheral conversion of androstenedione accounts for the rest.

Conclusion

The significant differences in the steroid profile between the premenopausal and the postmenopausal female are therefore as follows:

1. The blood production rates of estrogen decrease.
2. The cyclicity of estrogen production is lost.
3. Cyclic production of progesterone ceases.
4. There is an increase in the plasma levels of androgens relative to the reduction in estrogen values.
5. The major free estrogen becomes estrone, with about 40 μg per day being excreted.
6. Androstenedione becomes of considerable importance as a precursor of estrone although it is still uncertain what factors actually influence peripheral conversion. Initially, the ovary and adrenal are the major sources of androstenedione, and estrone production remains fairly constant. Eventually, with age, the ovarian stroma will cease production. The adrenal contribution, inadequate as a single source, will not be able to maintain sufficient estrone production, and specific target-tissue deficiencies will become apparent.

One final important piece of information should be added. It may be that not all postmenopausal women are the same, and the differences may be in the ovaries. Procope has clearly shown two populations of postmenopausal females to exist. One group demonstrated atrophic ovaries after menopause and oophorectomy makes little difference to steroid production. The second group showed ovarian cortical stromal hyperplasia, and removal of these ovaries makes a considerable difference to the postoperative steroid profile.[36]

PITUITARY GONADOTROPINS AND RELEASING FACTORS

The alterations that occur in hypothalamic-pituitary function before, during, and after menopause are, by all indications, purely secondary responses to the events in the ovary itself. Thus the hypothalamic-pituitary mechanism remains essentially intact after menopause and able to respond to fluctuating sex steroid levels, whether endogenous or exogenous.

Estrogens are known to be formed, bound, and biologically active in specific areas of rat brain, and determine a variety of functional and anatomic changes in neuronal wiring at the synaptic level.[37] It is interesting to speculate whether early programming of the hypothalamic-pituitary mechanism in the human fetus and child will determine later responses at menopause. For the moment, such matters rest in the area of pure theory and will not be alluded to again.

Another developing area in hypothalamic neurochemistry is that of catecholestrogen metabolism. Hypothalamic tissue concentrations of catecholestrogens, that is, those estrogens metabolized at the carbon-2 position to methoxy- and other hydroxyestrogens (2-hydroxy-estrogen), are at least ten times higher than those of their parent compounds.[38] These compounds may therefore have an important role in neuroendocrine regulation.

Perimenopausal

Before menopause, pituitary gonadotropin production and release is governed by two centers in the hypothalamus. The tonic center is responsible for a basal production of FSH and LH, while the cyclic center responds to actual demand by an acute release of FSH and LH. These centers are themselves influenced by the ovarian steroids, estradiol, estrone, and progesterone. A positive or negative feedback will be induced, depending on how these steroids occupy receptor sites in the hypothalamus, and this will be reflected as an increase or decrease in GnRH production.

The changes in ovarian steroid profiles around menopause, as previously discussed, profoundly influence this delicate mechanism. These changes precede menopause, when positive and negative feedback mechanisms are slightly altered but still present. After menopause, the cyclicity of these mechanisms disappears.

The first detectable endocrine manifestation of reproductive aging is a gradual increase in plasma FSH levels. This rise becomes apparent almost a decade before menopause, despite apparently normal ovulatory cycles.[17,18,21,23] Although this change has been demonstrated as early as age 34, it only becomes statistically significant at about 40 to 44 years of age.[17]

Sometime after the FSH level increases, there is a concomitant increase in serum LH levels, usually at age 45 to 50. The possibility that these changes may be induced by marginal decreases in estradiol production were discussed earlier.[18,23]

Further theories have been postulated for this early elevation in FSH. Sherman and Korenman[18,23] have suggested that an ovarian follicular substance may exist which could selectively suppress FSH secretion. Analagous to the testicular inhibin of the male, the name *FSH-release inhibiting substance* (FRIS) has been suggested.[39] Considerable support has developed for this theory.[17,39] Moreover, the recent finding of inhibin-like activity in bovine follicular fluid[40] does make the idea attractive that a progressive decline in number of ovarian follicles could result in reduced production of inhibin, and a concomitant rise in FSH levels in postmenopausal women. Such a substance has recently been purified from human ovarian follicular fluid.[40A]

Another theory to explain the premenopausal increase in FSH production is the possibility of an age-related change in the hypothalamo-pituitary sensitivity to feedback inhibition by ovarian steroids. Finally, it is possible that there is a progressive reduction in ovarian responsiveness to gonadotropin stimulation. Support for the latter theory comes from the observation that older premenopausal women need higher doses of gonadotropins for induction of ovulation.[41]

Postmenopausal

GONADOTROPINS   After the menopause, the elevation in blood levels of both FSH and LH is quite dramatic.[42] Indeed, there is a fourteen-fold increase of FSH compared to the premenopausal state,[43] and over a three-fold increase in LH.[44] The levels of both gonadotropins in the circulation reach a maximum at about two to three years after spontaneous menopause.[45]

The difference between the FSH and the LH increase led to the suggestion that the LH/FSH ratio could be used as a means to determine whether the patient is postmenopausal. Lauritzen studied the ratio of LH to FSH in peripheral venous blood before and after bilateral oophorectomy, finding the value to change from >1 to <0.7 in four days after castration. He felt that an LH/FSH ratio of less than 0.7 indicated ovarian failure.[42] Others have found the ratio of LH to FSH to vary from 0.6 to 2.3.[45] Although this suggests the index to be of little additional diagnostic value, the significant increase in FSH is in itself a diagnostic criterion of menopause.

The FSH and LH values, following their peak at about 3 years postmenopause, gradually decline over the next 30 years to values of some 40 to 50 percent of these maximal levels.[45] The actual values are shown in Table 3-2.

The hypothalamic-pituitary mechanism responds extremely rapidly to removal of both ovaries from a premenopausal woman. These responses are preceded by a more rapid decrease in the plasma estradiol level. FSH levels are significantly elevated by day two and LH by day three, as compared to preoperative control values.[32] The phase of the

Table 3-2. Mean Concentration of Plasma FSH and LH in Postmenopausal Women

| | Years After Menopause | | | | | |
	1	2-3	5	10	20	30
FSH (IU/ml)	48	66	55	42	27	24
LH (IU/ml)	54	61	48	55	29	30

Adapted from Chakravarti et al.: Br Med J 2:784, 1976

cycle in which surgery is performed does modify these responses
slightly.[46]

RELEASING FACTORS   The ability to measure the gonadotropin
releasing hormones in plasma involves a technique of recent origin.
Moreover, the amounts of peripheral plasma probably only indirectly
reflect the amounts or activity in the hypothalamic-hypophyseal portal
system. At the present time, little information is available as a result of
the difficulties involved in human investigation in this area.

LRH concentration has been reported to be higher in postmenopause and these concentrations do appear to correspond to LH levels.[47]
Lauritzen was unable to confirm these findings, although a periodic
release of LRH was demonstrated.[42]

It is of interest that the intravenous administration of LRH to
postmenopausal women provokes an additional very high increase in the
plasma levels of FSH and LH.[42] Thus there would appear to be a reserve
capacity for additional release of FSH and LH despite the already-
existing high pituitary production of these hormones. These findings are
evidence of the intactness of the hypothalamic-anterior pituitary
system after the menopause.

PROLACTIN

There is a remarkable amount of information becoming available
about prolactin, particularly as it is less than a decade since human prolactin was isolated.[48] There is a significant correlation between circulating prolactin levels and estradiol levels during the menstrual cycle and
the postmenopausal period.[17,48] Thus in women there is an increase in
prolactin after puberty and a decrease after menopause. Estrogen and
prolactin levels appear to run parallel to each other. A stimulatory effect of pharmacologic amounts of exogenous estrogen upon prolactin
secretion tends to support the evidence for this relationship.[49]

Hyperprolactinemia and its relationship to the reproductive processes is presently under intense scrutiny. With regard to menopause, however, current thinking is that the low estrogen levels are responsible for the lowered overall prolactin secretion.[50] Certainly, around menopause ovarian inactivity is not related to hyperprolactinemia.[48]

There is no information as to what the changes in prolactin levels produce in terms of target tissue responses. Membrane receptors for prolactin have been found in many tissues including breast, gonads, liver, and kidney.[48]

GONADOTROPIN AND SEX STEROID RESPONSE TO EXOGENOUS HORMONES

Despite widespread clinical usage of exogenous estrogens and progestins, there is unfortunately a remarkable lack of reported studies concerning the effect of such therapy on the endogenous hormone profiles. Furthermore, refinement of laboratory techniques to prevent grossly excessive cross-reactions to related immunoreactive hormones, as well as the ability to measure different and previously immeasurable substances, creates the need to repeat many studies done five years ago or longer.

There is a distinct need for information on the effects of exogenous hormones on the endogenous hormone profiles. Since normal menopause and oophorectomy are associated with specific changes in hormone profile, reflected in target tissue changes to be discussed in the next chapter, there are claims that hormone replacement will prevent or reverse such effects. The question that immediately arises is whether the normal premenopausal hormone profiles can be reproduced in the postmenopausal female by the use of such exogenous hormones. The answer to date appears negative, but, as mentioned, the information is limited.

Gonadotropin Response

Tsai and Yen studied the acute effects of an intravenous infusion of 17 β-estradiol on gonadotropin release in postmenopausal women. There was a significant and rapid decline of FSH and LH after infusion of 17 β-estradiol.[51] It does not appear, however, as if exogenous estrogens in dosages elevating estrogens to normal premenopausal levels are at the same time able to reduce gonadotropin levels to their average premenopausal values. Thus the short-term effect of micronized

17 β-estradiol, for example, is to produce marked increases in serum concentrations of E_1 and E_2, and depressions of gonadotropin levels, but not to premenopausal levels in the case of the latter.[52] Estradiol implants after oophorectomy, however, have been reported to prevent the expected rise in gonadotropins that would occur after castration.[53]

In light of the above discrepancies, the following information is of interest. Utian et al. measured FSH, LH, and estradiol (E_2) serially in premenopausal patients before and after oophorectomy, and following incremental doses of conjugated estrogens, with each dose interspersed by two weeks without therapy.[32] In only one instance did the exogenous estrogen succeed in reducing FSH to premenopausal levels (Figure 3-1). This was at a dosage of 2.5 mg, in which instance the E_2 level was higher than the premenopausal value (Figure 3-2). LH was never reduced to a premenopausal level (Figure 3-3).

Similar findings were reported by Lauritzen, who concluded that complete suppression doses for FSH and LH would have to be in excess of 6 to 8 mg estrone sulfate per day.[42] This would be a grossly excessive dose in terms of the effect on plasma estrogen levels.

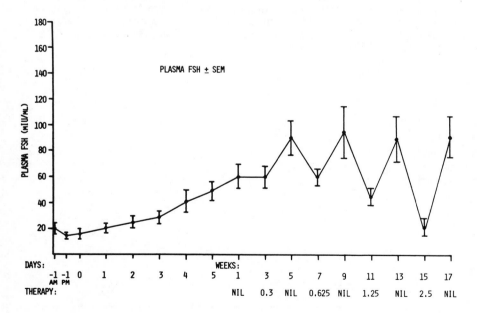

Figure 3-1.   Mean plasma FSH levels before and after surgery and following incremental doses of conjugated estrogens, interspersed by treatment-free periods. (From Utian et al.: Am J Obstet Gynecol 132:207, 1978. Courtesy of C V Mosby Co.).

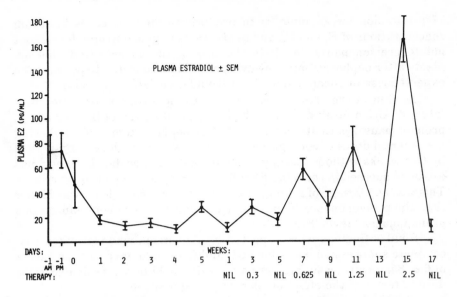

Figure 3-2.　Mean plasma estradiol (E_2) levels before and after surgery and following incremental doses of conjugated estrogens, interspersed by treatment-free periods. (From Utian et al.: Am J Obstet Gynecol 132:297, 1978. Courtesy of C.V. Mosby Co.).

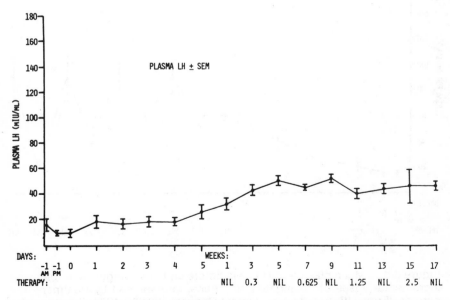

Figure 3-3.　Mean plasma LH levels before and after surgery and following incremental doses of conjugated estrogens, interspersed by treatment-free periods. (From Utian et al.: Am J Obstet Gynecol 132:297, 1978. Courtesy of C V Mosby Co.).

It is therefore appropriate at this time to conclude it unlikely that any single dose of exogenous estrogen will elevate E_2 levels to the mean premenopausal value and yet at the same time reduce FSH and LH levels to their premenopausal means. Of course, the question as to whether this maneuver is necessary or beneficial also remains to be proven.[32]

Sex Steroid Response

A number of groups have investigated the effects of exogenous estrogen therapy on steroid hormone levels.[32,52-56] Conjugated estrogens (CE) readily increase the circulating levels of E_1 and E_2.[53] To obtain a plasma E_2 level after oophorectomy that is similar to the premenopausal value, a dosage of CE of no less than 0.625 mg per day and no more than 1.25 mg per day is required (Figure 3-2).[32]

There appears to be little doubt that, following administration, the orally-ingested estrogens undergo rapid conversion, possibly in the gastrointestinal tract. Thus the plasma estrogen fractions may bear little resemblance to the formula of the tablet taken.[56] For instance, oral tablets of estradiol valerate and piperazine estrone sulfate result in virtually identical concentrations of E_1, E_2, and E_2 sulfate.[56] This is an important finding as it tends to discredit the estrone hypothesis in the etiology of endometrial cancer,[57] suggesting that the excess risk of endometrial carcinoma applies to systemic estrogens of various kinds and not only to conjugated equine estrogens.

The effects of exogenous estrogens have also been evaluated for effects on adrenal steroids. Thus far it would appear that administered estrogens have only a limited effect on adrenocortical steroidogenesis, although they do increase the concentration of transcortin.[55]

The effect of adding progestins to the estrogen therapy regime remains to be clarified. When administered in combination as in the oral contraceptive, a significant suppression of estradiol is observed in association with a great increase in serum and urine androgen concentrations.[58] This finding raises the suspicion that the combination oral contraceptive pill could produce a state of "pseudomenopause," certainly from the blood steroid profile point of view anyway. The ultimate outcome of these steroid alterations on target tissues also remains to be evaluated.

CONCLUSION

Loss of ovarian function, spontaneous or otherwise, is associated with profound alterations in the patterns of gonadotropin and sex steroid hormone production, metabolism, and clearance. Administration of exogenous hormones in turn influences these factors. In some instances the postmenopausal profile can be reversed to the premenopausal situation; in other instances new patterns are created, the significance of which is ill understood. The fact that the postmenopause is more than a time of estrogen deficiency, however, needs little further emphasis.

The changes in hormone concentrations will ultimately be reflected in selective responses on target tissues in which these hormones have specific receptor sites. It is these target tissue changes that will be considered in the next chapter.

References

1.   Reid DE, Ryan KJ, Benirshke K: Principles and Management of Human Reproduction. Philadelphia, Saunders, 1972

2.   Lloyd CW, Lobotsky J, Baird DT, et al: Concentration of unconjugated estrogens, androgens and gestogens in ovarian and peripheral venous plasma of women: the menstrual cycle. J Clin Endocrinol Metab 32:155, 1971

3.   Baird DT, Fraser IS: Blood production and ovarian secretion rates of estradiol-17B and estrone in women throughout the menstrual cycle. J Clin Endocrinol Metab 38:1009, 1974

4.   Loraine JA, Bell ET: Hormone Assays and Their Clinical Application. Baltimore, Williams and Wilkins, 1971

5.   Tait JF: Review: The use of isotopic steroids for the measurement of production rates *in vivo*. J Clin Endocrinol Metab 23:1285, 1963

6.   Longcope C, Kato T, Horton R: Conversion of blood androgens to estrogens in normal adult men and women. J Clin Invest 48:2191, 1969

7.   Grodin JM, Siiteri PK, MacDonald PC: Source of estrogen production in postmenopausal women. J Clin Endocrinol Metab 36:307, 1973

8.   Longcope C: Metabolic clearance and blood production rates of estrogens in postmenopausal women. Am J Obstet Gynecol 111:778, 1971

9.   Taylor RW: Estrogen target organs and receptor. In Cambell S (ed): The Management of the Menopause. Baltimore, University Park Press, 1976, p 97

10.   Jensen EV, Suzuki T, Numata M, Smith S, de Sombre ER: Estrogen-binding substances in target tissues. Steroids 13:417, 1969

11.   Rochefort H, Lignon F, Capony F: Formation of estrogen nuclear receptor in uterus: Effect of androgens, estrone and nafoxidine. Biochem Biophys Res Commun 47:662, 1972

12.   Mishell DR, Nakamura RM, Grosignani PG, et al.: Serum gonadotropin and steriod patterns during the normal menstrual cycle. Am J Obstet Gynecol 111:60, 1971

13.   Baird DT, Horton R, Longcope C, et al.: Steroid dynamics under steady-state conditions. Recent Prog Horm Res 25:611, 1969

14.   Mikhail G: Hormone secretion by the human ovary. Gynecol Invest 1:5, 1970

15.   Kirschner MA, Jacobs JF: Combined ovarian and adrenal vein catheterization to determine the site(s) of androgen overproduction in hirsute women. J Clin Endocrinol Metab 33:199, 1971

16.   Treloar AE, Boynton RE, Benn BG, Brown BW: Variation of the human menstrual cycle through reproductive life. Int J Fertil 12:77, 1967

17.   Reyes FI, Winter SD, Faiman C: Pituitary-ovarian relationships preceding the menopause. Am J Obstet Gynecol 129:557, 1977

18.   Sherman BM, Korenman SG: Hormonal characteristics of the human menstrual cycle throughout reproductive life. J Clin Invest 55:699, 1975

19.   Furuhjelm M: Urinary excretion of hormones during the climacteric. Acta Obstet Gynecol Scand 45:352, 1966

20.   England P K, Skinner LG, Cottrell KM, Sellwood RA: Serum oestradiol-17 β in normal women. Br J Cancer 29:462, 1974

21.   Wide L, Nillius SJ, Gemzell C, Roos P: Radio immunoabsorbent assay of FSH and LH in serum and urine from men and women. Acta Endocrinol Suppl 174:41, 1973

22.   Pincus G, Romanoff LP, Carlo J: The excretion of urinary steroids by men and women of various ages. J Gerontol 9:113, 1954

23.   Sherman BM, West JH, Korenman SG: The menopausal transition: Analysis of LH, FSH, estradiol and progesterone concentrations during menstrual cycles of older women. J Clin Endocrinol Metab 42:247, 1976

24.   Papanicolaou AD, Loraine JA, Dove GA, Loudon NB: Hormone excretion patterns in perimenopausal women. J Obstet Gynaecol Br Cwlth 76:308, 1969

25.   Poliak A, Jones GES, Goldberg B, Woodruff JD: Effect of human chorionic gonadotrophin on postmenopausal women. Am J Obstet Gynecol 101:731, 1968

26.   Hensell DL, Grodin JM, Brennet PF, Siiteri PK, MacDonald PC: Plasma precursors of estrogens. II Correlation of the extent of conversion of plasma androstenedione to estrone with age. J Clin Endocrinol Metab 38:476, 1974

27.   MacDonald PC, Edman CD, Hemsell DL, Porter JC, Siiteri PK: Effect of obesity on conversion of plasma androstenedione to estrone in postmenopausal women with and without endometrial cancer. Am J Obstet Gynecol 130:448, 1978

28.   Thijssen JHH, Longcope C: Postmenopausal estrogen production. In van Keep PA (ed): Consensus on Menopause Research. Lancaster, MTP Press, 1976, p 25

29.   Judd HL, Lucas WE, Yen SSC: Effect of oophorectomy on circulating testosterone and androstenedione levels in patients with endometrial cancer. Am J Obstet Gynecol 118:793, 1974

30.   Judd HL, Judd GE, Lucas WE, Yen SSC: Endocrine function of the postmenopausal ovary: concentrations of androgens and estrogens in ovarian and peripheral vein blood. J Clin Endocrinol Metab 39:1020, 1974

31.   Hammond CB: Menopause, an American view. In Campbell S (ed): Management of the Menopause. Baltimore, University Park Press, 1976, p 405

32.   Utian WH, Katz M, Davey DA, Carr PJ: Effect of premenopausal castration and incremental dosages of conjugated equine estrogens on plasma FSH, LH and estradiol. Am J Obstet Gynecol 132:297, 1978

33.   Vermeulen A: The hormonal activity of the postmenopausal ovary. J Clin Endocrinol Metab 42:247, 1976

34.   Horton R, Tait JF: Androstenedione production and interconversion rates measured in peripheral blood and studies on the possible site of its conversion to testosterone. J Clin Invest 45:301, 1966

35.   Bardin CW, Lipsett MB: Testosterone and androstenedione blood production rates in normal women and women with idiopathic hirsutism or polycystic ovaries. J Clin Invest 46:891, 1967

36.   Procope B: Studies on the urinary excretion, biological effects and origin of oestrogens in postmenopausal women. Acta Endocrinol Suppl 135:1, 1968

37.   Naftolin F, Brewer JR: The effect of estrogens on hypothalamic structure and function. Am J Obstet Gynecol 132:758, 1978

38.   Paul SM, Axelrod J: Catechol estrogens: presence in brain and endocrine tissues. Science 197:657, 1977

39.   van Look PFA, Lothian H, Hunter WM, Michie EA, Baird ST: Hypothalamic-pituitary-ovarian function in perimenopausal women. Clin Endocrinol 7:13, 1977

40.   De Jong FH, Sharpe RM: Evidence of inhibin-like activity in bovine follicular fluid. Nature 263:71, 1976

40A.   Chari S, Hopkinson CRN, Daume E, Sturm G: Purification of INHIBIN from human ovarian follicular fluid. Acta Endocrinol (Kbh) 90:157, 1979

41.   Van de Wiele, Bogumil J, Dyrenfurth I, et al.: Mechanisms regulating the menstrual cycle in women. Recent Prog Horm Res 26:63, 1970

42.   Lauritzen C: The hypothalamic anterior pituitary system in the climacteric age period. In Estrogens in the Post-menopause. Front Horm Res 3:20, Basel, Karger, 1975

43.   Coble YD, Kohler PO, Cargille CM, Ross GT: Production rates and metabolic clearance rates of human FSH in premenopausal and postmenopausal women. J Clin Invest 48:539, 1969

44.   Kohler PO, Ross GT, Odell WD: Metabolic clearance and production rates of human luteinizing hormone in pre- and post-menopausal women. J Clin Invest 47:38, 1968

45.   Chakravarti S, Collins WP, Forecast JD, et al.: Hormonal profiles after the menopause. Br Med J 2:784, 1976

46.   Yen SSC, Tsai CC: The effect of ovariectomy on gonadotropin release. J Clin Invest 50:1149, 1971

47.   Seyler LE, Reichlin S: Luteinizing hormone-releasing factor (LRF) in plasma of postmenopausal women. J Clin Endocrinol Metab 37:197, 1973

48.   Ben-David M, L'Hermite M: Prolactin and menopause. In van Keep PA (ed): Consensus on Menopause Research. Lancaster, MTP Press, 1976, p 19

49.   Yen SSC, Ehara Y, Siler TM: Augmentation of prolactin secretion by estrogen in hypogonadal women. J Clin Invest 53:652, 1974

50.   Vekemans M, Robyn C: Influence of age on serum prolactin in women and men. Br Med J 4:738, 1975

51.   Tsai CC, Yen SSC: Acute effects of intravenous infusion of 17B-estradiol on gonadotropin release in pre- and postmenopausal women. J Clin Endocrinol 32:766, 1971

52.   Yen SSC, Martin PL, Burnier AM, et al.: Circulating estradiol, estrone and gonadotropin levels following the administration of orally active 17B-estradiol in postmenopausal women. J Clin Endocrinol Metab 40:518, 1975

53.   Hunter DJS, Julier D, Franklin M, Green E: Plasma levels of estrogen, LH and FSH following castration and estradiol implant. Obstet Gynecol 49:180, 1976

54.   Rose DP, Fern M, Liskowski L, Milbrath JR: Effect of treatment with estrogen conjugates on endogenous plasma steroids. Obstet Gynecol 49:80, 1977

55.   Mahajan DK, Billiar RB, Jassani M, Little AB: Ethinyl estradiol administration and plasma steroid concentrations in ovariectomized women. Am J Obstet Gynecol 130:398, 1978

56.   Anderson ABM, Sklovsky E, Sayers L Steele PA, Turnbull AC: Comparison of serum oestrogen concentrations in post-menopausal women taking oestrone sulphate and oestradiol. Br Med J 1:140, 1978

57.   Siiteri PK, Schwartz BE, MacDonald PC: Estrogen receptors and the estrone hypothesis in relation to endometrial and breast cancer. Gynecol Oncol 2:228, 1974

58.   Kjeld JM, Puah CM, Joplin GF: Changed levels of endogenous sex steroids in women on oral contraceptives. Br Med J 2:1354, 1976

4

Target Tissue Response to Ovarian Failure

In view of the fact that the menopause occurs at a time of life when there is a rising incidence of degenerative disease, it is not surprising that a causal relationship between some of these degenerative disorders and climacteric endocrine changes should have been postulated. Proof of a direct relationship is generally lacking between estrogen deprivation and development of any particular metabolic derangement or degenerative process. In some instances, indirect evidence has been produced. Moreover, despite an intense interest generated in recent years over the metabolic effects of perimenopausal ovarian failure, little is yet known about how steroids act at the cellular level in postmenopausal women. The purpose of the present chapter is to outline those specific tissue alterations most likely related to the endocrinologic changes outlined in Chapter 3.

TARGET ORGANS AND SEX STEROID ACTION

Sex steroid synthesis, release, and receptor uptake has been described in Chapter 3. Target tissues were defined as being tissues characterized by the presence of highly specific protein receptor molecules within the cells that are able to bind firmly to the specific circulating steroid. As a result of the presence of these specific receptors, target tissues can be triggered into action by the hormones which circulate in very low concentrations.

The absence of a specific hormone receptor in a tissue would result, theoretically at least, in that tissue being immune to the relevant hormone effect. It is possible, however, that a tissue may be indirectly affected by changes in the endocrinologic profile. For example, until now no estrogen receptors have been demonstrated to be present in osseous tissue, although ovarian function appears to have a definite effect on bone resorption. In this instance, estrogens may indirectly affect osseous tissue by a direct effect on parathyroid hormone function (see Chapter 5).

Receptors have been identified in many tissues, including ovary, endometrium, vaginal epithelium, and hypothalamus. These tissues will thus respond to the presence or absence of steroid hormones by definitive alterations in structure or function. It is these peripheral target tissue responses that are of interest in this chapter.

The actual mechanism by which the steroids influence the gene activity is largely unknown, but information in this respect is developing at an exciting pace.[1-4] Although an in-depth consideration of this mechanism goes beyond the bounds of this monograph, the best documented aspects of sex steroid action in reproductive organs are worth listing.[5]

1. The cell membrane does not act as a selective barrier to the entry of steroid hormones. Thus the hormones freely diffuse across the cell membrane.

2. Each target cell contains about 10,000 receptor molecules. These will selectively bind the specific steroid, and result in a relatively greater concentration of the steroid in the specific target tissue as compared to nontarget tissues which lack these receptors.[5]

3. The actual number or level of receptors in the target tissue cell can vary. For example, 17 beta-estradiol induces its own receptors; that is, it influences the level of 17 beta-estradiol-specific receptors. This process is called *replenishment*. Thus the measure of cytoplasmic estradiol receptors increases in estradiol-exposed target tissues such as uterus and vagina, or becomes less in nonexposed tissues.[6,7] From a clinical standpoint this would explain an increasing response to prolonged hormonal therapy.

4. Hormones can also increase the concentration of receptors for other hormones. For example, estradiol will not only increase its own receptors, but can increase target tissue responsiveness to progesterone by increasing the intracellular receptors for progesterone.

5. The steroid-receptor complex passes within minutes from the cytoplasm to the nucleus, and the resultant chromatin bound sex-steroid receptor then appears to remain in the nucleus for several hours even though the sex steroids may be withdrawn. Complex genome (RNA synthesis) activity is then initiated.[1,2,3,4] Thus the hormone-receptor complex binds to nuclear DNA resulting in synthesis of messenger RNA (mRNA). The mRNA is transported to the ribosomes.

6. The above activity will result in new protein formation that is specific for the target tissue and gene that is activated. For instance, cervical glandular cells will be induced to produce cervical mucus whereas vaginal cells will be stimulated to undergo maturation processes.

7. It is distinctly possible that different tissues may respond differently to various estrogenic agents.[8] Alternatively, it may be possible in the future that steroid analogues can be developed that have the

property of maintaining the differentiated characteristics of the actual target tissue without inducing further and undesired cellular proliferation.[9]

In summary, there are four essential factors responsible for hormonal activity and biologic response:

1. The circulating concentration of the free hormone (as opposed to the bound)
2. The concentration of receptors
3. The dissociation rate of the hormone-receptor complex
4. The dissociation rate of the hormone-receptor complex bound to the chromatin

A fifth factor is sometimes necessary; that is, intracellular hormone conversion. For example, testosterone may need to be converted to dihydrotestosterone in the cell before being able to initiate the above reaction.

The specific pelvic and extrapelvic target tissues will now be considered individually in terms of their response to ovarian function and its ultimate failure at the climacteric.

PELVIC ORGANS

The sex steroid hormone-related changes in each of the major pelvic structures of importance will be described in the following order:

1. Normal anatomy
2. Response to endogenous sex steroids during the reproductive years
3. Response to altered hormonal profiles during and after the climacteric

Vulva

STRUCTURE   Although *vulva* is a composite term for the external genitalia (mons pubis, labia majora and minora, clitoris, vaginal opening, hymen, and vestibule), common usage also includes the Bartholin's glands and the perineum. The skin of the mons pubis and labia majora contain hair follicles, sebaceous glands, and sweat glands, including specialized apocrine glands. The skin of the labia minora is smooth, containing sebaceous glands but no hair follicles and few, if any, sweat glands. The labia minora and the clitoris, or penile homologue, are richly vascular, allowing for a turgid response to sexual stimulation, and have an extensive nerve supply for the same reason. The Bartholin's glands, one on each side of the posterolateral orifice of the vagina, are racemose in type and lobulated. The glandular acini are lined by simple columnar or cuboidal epithelium responsible for a colorless, mucoid secretion, produced essentially as a lubricant following on sexual excitement.

RESPONSE TO AGING   The vulval structures show a striking response to age, hormonal environment, and sexual functions. The labia are small, particularily the labia minora, until adolescence, and the mons pubis and labia majora are devoid of hair. With adolescence there is deposition of fat in the mons pubis and labia majora, and pubic hair growth usually precedes the onset of menstruation by at least two years. The increase in size of the labia majora invariably results in the labia minora and vaginal orifice becoming hidden.

Sexual intercourse, pregnancy, and childbirth produce a number of changes in the vulva. Stretching or tearing of the perineum usually results in it becoming shorter, making the vaginal orifice appear wider and more exposed. Following menopause the vulval structures gradually undergo atrophy. Hair loss is progressive, and the skin becomes thinner, often in old age having a glazed or shiny appearance. The subcutaneous tissues all but disappear so that the labia majora become very small and the labia minora almost nonexistent. Dystrophies and pruritis of the vulva are much more frequent in postmenopausal women.

Vagina

STRUCTURE   The vagina is a fibromuscular canal that demonstrates remarkable elasticity. By correct terminology the lining of the vagina is an epithelium rather than a mucosa because it does not contain any glands. So-called "vaginal secretion" is really a result of breakdown of superficial cells. The "sweating phenomenon" of sexual intercourse, however, may represent a transudate.[10] It is worth emphasizing that the vagina is capable to a very high degree of absorption of water, electrolytes, and substances of low molecular weight. Local medicaments such as estrogen creams will thus be absorbed and can have systemic effects.

The vaginal epithelium is made up of four distinct layers:

1. The *basal layer* rests directly on the fibromuscular tissues and is the source of the continous production of the cells comprising the layers above.
2. Next is the *parabasal layer* which represents a maturation of the basal cells.

3. The *intermediate layer* can be differentiated from the deeper cells by the presence of glycogen, which can be confirmed by a brown stain with the application of iodine.
4. The *superficial layer* represents a final differentiation at the surface. Keratinization does not occur under normal circumstances, but can follow exposure of the vagina to air as in the case of severe vaginal prolapse.

VAGINAL CYTOLOGY

The vaginal cells can be differentiated on stained vaginal smears. Despite the fact that this has been known for years[11] (or perhaps because of it) there is a diversity of terms and definitions used for the cells that desquamate from this squamous epithelium. These have been well reviewed,[12,13] and for the purpose of this discussion are correctly defined as follows:[14-16]

1. Parabasal cells are determined on a basis of cellular size, the limits being a diameter of 15-30 μ, and shape, the cells demonstrating a round or oval circumference with no angulation.
2. Intermediate cells are identified as squamous cells presenting a definite differentiation of cytoplasm, a beginning retraction of the nuclear diameter, but without complete karyopyknosis.
3. Superficial cells are distinguished from other cells above all by their pyknotic nucleus, which is defined as one which does not exceed 5.5μ in diameter and appears black and structureless.

The actual differentiation of parabasal from intermediate and superficial cells is fairly straightforward. Separating intermediate from superficial cells is more difficult. Wied suggested the use of phase-contrast microscopy for this purpose because pyknotic nuclei shine a brilliant red as compared to the darker, more opaque appearance of non-pyknotic nuclei.[17]

A number of hormonal indices have been described based on the varying ratios of these cells present on a lateral fornix smear. Much has been made of these indices in relation to menopausal therapy, to the extent that often the smear rather than the patient is being treated. Unfortunately, these cytologic indices of hormonal function are of relatively limited value when globally assessed in groups of patients because they vary from patient to patient. In fact, in individual patients their value is enhanced by serial smear evaluation, and the interpretation of single smears may be difficult.

The actual *cytologic indices* often used include the following:

1. *Maturation index* (MI). This represents the ratio of parabasal, intermediate and superficial cells present on the smear expressed as a percentage (e.g., 9 parabasals: 91 intermediates: 0 superficials).

2. *Karyopyknotic index* (KPI). This represents the ratio of superficial cells to intermediate cells.
3. *Eosinophilic index* (EI). This represents the ratio of mature eosinophilic cells to mature cyanophilic cells.
4. *Folded cell index* (FCI). This represents the ratio of folded mature cells to flat mature cells.

For further details about the use of the vaginal smear in evaluating female hormonal status, the reader is referred to an excellent review by Wied and Bibbo.[13] In actual fact, however, there are only two diagnostic cell patterns:

1. The *estrogenic pattern.* Estrogenic stimulation is confirmed by a vaginal smear showing mature, separate-lying cells, some of which are superficial and the rest intermediate in type.
2. The *atrophic pattern.* A cell pattern consisting essentially of intermediate and parabasal-type cells is diagnostic of a nonestrogen stimulated vaginal epithelium.

Utian has recommended the use of a *parabasal cell index* to define the estrogenic status of postmenopausal females.[18] This is simply the percentage of parabasal cells present on a vaginal smear. Estrogens cause the disappearance of the parabasal cells from the vaginal smear (Figure 4-1).

RESPONSE TO AGING   In simple terms the presence of estrogen stimulates the maturation of the vaginal epithelium from the basal layers through to the superficial layer. This explains the cytologic picture previously described. The absence of estrogen stimulation results in lack of epithelial growth, confirmed by the presence of parabasal cells on the vaginal smear.

During reproductive age, the vaginal epithelium demonstrates a cyclic response parallel to the changing endocrine profile. Glycogen rich cells are produced which are acted upon by the Doderleins bacilli with the production of lactic acid and a resultant vaginal pH of 4.0 to 5.5.[10]

Regular intercourse results in some stretching of the vaginal walls, which is also aggravated by pregnancy and childbirth. The latter tends to reduce the number of vaginal rugae, particularly if there is uterovaginal prolapse.

The vagina shows several specific responses to climacteric. Vaginal epithelial maturation decreases. There is a failure of production of the glycogen-containing superficial cells and ultimately an increase in vaginal pH to ranges between 6.0 and 8.0. The resistance of the vagina to pyogenic organisms becomes reduced, and a condition usually termed *atrophic vaginitis* may result. Even in the absence of this, the vagina

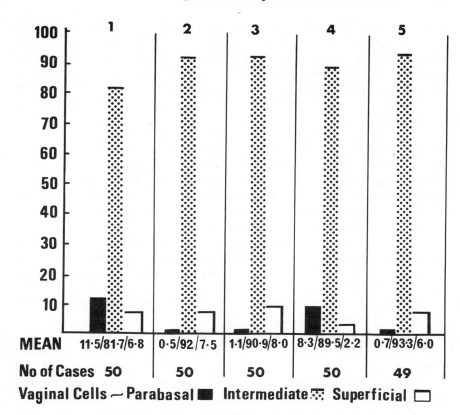

MEAN	11·5/81·7/6·8	0·5/92/7·5	1·1/90·9/8·0	8·3/89·5/2·2	0·7/93·3/6·0
No of Cases	50	50	50	50	49

Vaginal Cells — Parabasal ■ Intermediate ⠿ Superficial ☐

Figure 4–1.   Diagrammatic representation of change in Maturation Index induced by estrogen and placebo therapy. 1 = control; 2 = 3 months estradiol
valerate; 3 = 6 months estradiol valerate; 4 = placebo; 5 = 3 months conjugated estrogen therapy. The parabasal cell type shows the only statistically
significant difference (From Utian: S Afr Med J 44:69, 1970. Courtesy of South
African Medical Journal).

will tend to become shorter and narrower with obliteration of the
vaginal fornices and an eventual loss of vaginal rugae.

It should be emphasized that some of the above changes are prevented or slowed by the continuance of regular intercourse. This may be
due to purely mechanical reasons, or could be a result of absorption of
steroids from the ejaculate itself.

Uterus-Endometrium

STRUCTURE   The components of the uterus pertinent to this discussion are the *body* or *corpus* and the *cervix*. The muscular component
of the uterine wall, or *myometrium,* is comprised of two layers. The in-

ner layer forms the bulk of the myometrium and is itself composed of involuntary muscle fibers which run obliquely in a watch-spring spiral fashion. The outer or superficial layer is continuous with the outer layers of the tubes and vagina and is composed of longitudinal fibers of involuntary muscle. Both layers also contain varying amounts of elastic and fibrous tissues in addition to the vascular, lymphatic, and nerve components.

The specialized uterine mucous membrane or *endometrium* rests directly on the muscular layer without intervening submucosa. Glands can therefore normally penetrate into the fibromuscular tissue of the myometrium. The endometrium is a single-layered cuboidal- or columnar-celled epithelium with simple (unbranched) spiral or tubular glands.

To the older woman particularly, the most important component of the cervix is the *endocervix* because of its malignant potentiality. The cervical muscous membrane is more complicated histologically than that of the uterus. The surface epithelium consists of tall columnar cells above a basal layer of cuboid cells. The glandular epithelium of the cervix is thicker than that of the endometrium and secretes an alkaline mucus, the constituents of which vary with the estrogenic status of the individual.

RESPONSE TO AGING   All of the uterine structures discussed above show specific changes with menarche, the reproductive cycle, and climacteric. In-depth descriptions of the menarchal and reproductive cycle changes are inappropriate here, and will not be dealt with further.

Following the climacteric the uterus becomes smaller and the walls thinner. The weight reduces from about 120 grams to 50 to 60 grams, and can be as little as 25 to 30 grams in advanced years.

The endometrium maintains the ability to respond to estrogenic stimulation. Normally it becomes cuboidal and thin, with short glands and fibrotic stroma, but it will proliferate following endogenous or exogenous estrogen stimulation. The relationship between endometrial hyperplasia, carcinoma and persistently raised blood estrogen concentrations will be dealt with in Chapter 9.

The perimenopausal alteration in hormone production results in an increased variability of menstrual cycle length. Prolonged intervals between menstrual periods are probably due to the shortage of follicles. Short cycles, however, may result either from a decrease in the length of the follicular phase,[19] or from defective luteal function.[20]

The cervix also shrinks after menopause with loss of the fornices, so that the external os is very nearly flush with the vaginal wall. The cervical mucus diminishes and eventually disappears. The endocervix becomes grossly atrophic and the cervical canal quite stenotic.

Fallopian Tube

The fallopian tube is functionally quiet after menopause. In essence the muscular and endosalpingeal changes in structure and function are similar to those of the uterus, and will not be discussed further.

Ovary

The structural and functional changes in the ovary itself were described in Chapters 2 and 3.

Bladder and Urethra

The bladder is a hollow muscular organ lined by transitional epithelium which is continuous with that of the urethra. This transitional epithelium demonstrates a similar response to ovarian hormones as does the vaginal epithelium. With aging, the bladder and urethra can be affected by atrophic cysto-urethritis, urethral caruncle, ectropion, and early stress incontinence.

Surprisingly, there is little valid documentation for an increase in stress incontinence and at least one good study to show little change in micturition patterns with advancing age.[21]

The distal urethra does appear to be sensitive to changing hormone profiles during the climacteric. This could result in atrophic distal-urethritis and structure formation, resulting in obstructive cystopathy with an increase in residual urine.[22] Ascending infection can be an inevitable result. Detrusor dysynergia is also a possible problem in such patients, although urethral pressure studies in menopausal patients on estrogens would suggest that more is involved than just the peri-urethral tissues.[23]

Much more information is necessary on the effects of climacteric on bladder and urethral function before any meaningful statements can be made about altered urodynamics after menopause.

The Pelvic Floor

STRUCTURE   The *pelvic floor* consists of all tissues lying between the pelvic cavity and the surface of the vulva and perineum.[10] This includes pelvic peritoneum, extraperitoneal fat and connective tissue, the levatores ani muscles and fascial coverings (*pelvic diaphragm*), the urogenital diaphragm, perineal muscles, and skin. The most important structures, however, are the levatores ani muscles, being voluntary muscles with several components supplied by the pudendal nerve and fibers directly from the S3 and S4 roots. Contraction of this musculature occurs in response to increased intra-abdominal pressure caused by coughing, sneezing, or similar strains.

RESPONSE TO AGING   The pelvic floor can become stretched or damaged following pregnancy and vaginal delivery. The muscular tissue of the pelvic floor appears to lose tone with decline of estrogen production. It is possible that the increased incidence of postmenopausal vaginal prolapse is probably related to tissue aging as much as to the alterations in hormone function and production. The ultimate effect of this combination of aging tissues and loss of hormonal stimulus is an increase in the incidence of cystocele, rectocele, enterocele, uterine prolapse, and combinations thereof.

EXTRAPELVIC EFFECTS

The hormonal changes after menopause or castration also appear to be associated with widespread effects on general target tissues or organs. Reports into direct etiologic relationships and mechanisms are still lacking in some specific areas, but information is beginning to accumulate about some organ system changes.

Skin

Of all the major body organs, skin best illustrates the difficulties in differentiating the general aging and environmental processes from the specific hormonal target tissue responses. Thus, skin, on the one hand, is a major hormone target tissue; on the other hand, it is one of the most abused body organs in terms of exposure to environmental hazards, particularly the sun. Both factors become cumulative from menopause onward.

ESTROGEN RECEPTORS   Estrogen receptors do exist in skin, although there is distinct need for precise identification.[24,25] Estrogens appear to have actions on all skin components and have been demonstrated to be actively bound and metabolized.[25,26]

EVALUATION OF SKIN   Distinct changes in the appearance of skin are difficult to scientifically document over a period of time. The fact that a man's skin differs from a woman's, or that a baby's differs from an adult's, is readily apparent. But how does one compare the skin of a forty-five-year-old woman to that of another aged fifty; or even to that of herself two or three years later? Therein lies the research difficulty, and the explanation for the sparsity of the literature in this respect. The following are some factors that are used experimentally:

1. Skin thickness
2. Number of mitoses
3. Degree of hyperemia or perfusion, measured by taking skin temperature or measuring perfusion by xenon clearance
4. Degree of water retention
5. Alteration of carbohydrate metabolism

Despite the difficulties in evaluation, there is information worthy of presentation.

SKIN CHANGES WITH AGE   The epidermis becomes progressively thinner after menopause. On microscopic section the epidermal ridges and dermal papillae become less prominent. Parallel with this change is a progressive decrease in the density of scalp and body hair follicles.[27] Sebaceous gland function appears to decline as well after loss of ovarian function.[28] Sweat glands also undergo a reduction in function and become less responsive to triggering stimuli.[29]

Diminution in sweat and sebaceous gland activity associated with epidermal thinning results in a dry, easily traumatized skin. This dryness will be aggravated in conditions of low humidity.[30] A usual complaint in this situation will be itching.

The dermis, too, becomes thinner, and several changes in collagen metabolism have been demonstrated. In particular, there are reduced amounts of soluble collagen with slower rates of collagen synthesis and turnover. There is, therefore, a reduced excretion of urinary hydroxyproline with age. Inevitably, there is a loss in the resilience and pliability of the skin.[30,31]

Evidence is beginning to accumulate that estrogen itself has a specific effect on collagen that can be differentiated from other biochemical effects.[9]

The mucous membranes also appear to be sensitive to ovarian function. Dry mouth, for example, has been described as a menopausal disorder.[32] Van Keep and Haspels feel that the voice also alters with a reduction in the upper register and a loss of timbre, hardly a problem to the average woman, but of potentially serious consequence for professional singers.[33]

In summary, therefore, it would appear from the limited information available that estrogens are actively bound and metabolized in all components of skin. Alteration in the function after menopause may contribute to the aging of skin by an effect additional to the concomitant aging process.

Cardiovascular System

Castration and normal climacteric appear to be related to change in blood-lipid profile, the development of atheromatosis, increase in hypertension, and the incidence of clinical coronary heart disease. There is not uniform agreement. This entire topic is discussed in depth in Chapter 6.

The Skeleton

Strong evidence exists to relate ovarian function to bone (osseous) metabolism. Castration or normal climacteric leads to negative calcium balance, increased bone resorption, osteoporosis, and an increased incidence of bone fracture. This subject is fully reviewed in Chapter 5.

Miscellaneous

BREASTS   One physical characteristic demonstrating a significant relationship to menopause and oophorectomy is that of breast configuration.[34] The mature breast undergoes cyclic changes during the normal reproductive cycle. Estrogen, growth hormone, and deoxycortone probably determine duct development, while glandular formation is under the influence of progesterone, prolactin, and the glucocorticoids.[10] Thus, in the luteal phase of the cycle there is increased epithelial activity which regresses during menstruation. Breast volume increases by as much as 100 ml in the second half of the menstrual cycle by a combination of glandular proliferation and water retention.[35] These cyclic changes explain the symptom production normally described during the reproductive cycle; for example, fullness or tenderness.

Following menopause the glandular tissue of the breast becomes atrophic. Breasts of thin women will thus tend to reduce in size and become flat, whereas those in obese women can remain large and pendulous. The breasts will also become atrophic following surgical castration.[34] This change would seem to occur fairly rapidly. Indeed, atrophy of the breasts becomes obvious as soon as six months after removal of functional ovaries from premenopausal women.[34]

The loss of elasticity in the Cooper's ligament aggravates the tendency of the breast to droop. The nipples become smaller and flatter, and lose their erectile properties.

THYROID FUNCTION   Changes may occur in thyroid function with age, but they are not sex-related. However, no definitive evidence seems to exist linking any change in thyroid function with menopause status. This is an unexpected finding in view of the profound effects that increased circulating estrogen levels, whether of exogenous or endogenous origin, have on thyroid function tests. The protein-bound iodine (PBI) increases with pregnancy or with exogenous estrogen administration, an effect due to an estrogen-induced increase in the binding proteins. However, thyroxine (T4) values tend to lie within relatively narrow limits during the normal reproductive cycle.[36] A reevaluation of thyroid status and menopausal status is probably worthwhile, although present indications are that failing ovarian function is unlikely to be associated with any dramatic change in thyroid status.

MOOD AND PSYCHOLOGIC STATUS   The relationship between ovarian function, menopause, oophorectomy and mental (psychic) status has proven extraordinarily difficult to evaluate. The differentiation between hormonally-induced symptoms from psychologic symptoms will be considered in Chapter 7.

CONCLUSION

A considerable amount of research is still necessary to define all the specific sites where sex-steroid hormone receptors may be present, and to clarify the response of these tissues to the altered endocrine state of climacteric. Nonetheless, more than enough evidence does exist to define the climacteric as an endocrinopathy in which alterations in hormonal profile are associated with extensive pelvic and extrapelvic target tissue effects. In general, these effects are of a negative nature that apparently hasten the general aging process.

References

1. Chan L, O'Malley BW: Mechanism of action of the sex steroid hormones. Part I. N Engl J Med 294:1322, 1976

2. Chan L, O'Malley BW: Mechanism of action of the sex steroid hormones. Part II. N Engl J Med 294:1372, 1976

3. Chan L, O'Malley BW: Mechanism of action of the sex steroid hormones. Part III. N Engl J Med 294:1430, 1976

4. Gorski J, Gannon F: Current models of steroid hormone action: a critique. Annu Rev Physiol 38:425, 1976

5. Finch CE, Flurkey K: The molecular biology of estrogen replacement. Contemp Obstet Gynecol 9:97, 1977

6. Pavlik EJ, Coulson PB: Modulation of estrogen receptors in four different target tissues: differential effects of estrogen and progesterone. J Steroid Biochem 7:369, 1976

7. Tsibris JCM, Cazenave CR, Cantor B, et al.: Distribution of cytoplasmic estrogen and progesterone receptors in human endometrium. Am J Obstet Gynecol 132:449, 1978

8. McPherson JC, Eldridge JC, Costoff A, Mahesh VB: The pituitary-gonadal axis before puberty: effects of various estrogenic steroids in the ovariectomized rat. Steroids 24:41, 1974

9. Meyer WJ, Henneman DH, Keiser HR, Bartter FC: 17 α-estradiol: separation of estrogen effect on collagen from other clinical and biochemical effects in man. Res Commun Chem Pathol Pharmacol 13:685, 1976

10. Jeffcoate N: Principles of Gynaecology, 4th ed. London, Butterworths, 1975

11. Papanicolaou OM, Traut HF: Diagnosis of Uterine Cancer by the Vaginal Smear. New York, The Commonwealth Fund, 1943

12. Gronroos M: Vaginal smear in postmenopause and its correlation with the urinary excretion of estrogens, 17-ketosteroids and gonadotropins. Acta Obstet Gynecol Scand 44, Suppl 5, 1, 1965

13. Wied GL, Bibbo M: Evaluation of endocrinologic condition by exfoliative cytology. In Gold JJ (ed): Textbook of Gynecologic Endocrinology, 2nd ed. Hagerstown, Md., Harper & Row, 1975

14. International Academy of Gynecological Cytology: Opinion poll on cytological definitions. Acta Cytol 2:26, 1958

15. de Neef JC: Clinical Endocrine Cytology. New York, Harper & Row, 1967

16. Wachtel EG: Exfoliative Cytology in Gynaecological Practice. London, Butterworths, 1964

17. Wied GL: Suggested standard for karyopyknosis: use in hormonal reading of vaginal smears. Fertil Steril 6:61, 1955

18. Utian WH: Use of vaginal smear in assessment of oestrogenic status of oophorectomized females. S Afr Med J 44:69, 1970

19. Van Look PFA, Lothian H, Hunter WM, et al.: Hypothalamic-pituitary-ovarian function in perimenopausal women. Clin Endocrinol 7:13, 1977

20. Sherman BM, Korenman SG: Hormonal characteristics of the human menstrual cycle throughout reproductive life. J Clin Invest 55:699, 1975

21. Osbourne JL: Post-menopausal changes in micturition habits and in urine flow and urethral pressure studies. In Campbell S (ed): Management of the Menopause. Baltimore, University Park Press, 1976, p 243

22. Smith PJB: The effect of estrogens on bladder function in the female. In Campbell S (ed): Management of the Menopause. Baltimore, University Park Press, 1976, p 291

23. Harrison RF: Urethral profile studies on menopausal women and the effects of estrogen treatment. In Campbell S (ed): Management of the Menopause. Baltimore, University Park Press, 1976, p 299

24. Frost P, Weinstein ED, Hsia SL: Metabolism of oestradiol and oestrone in human skin. J Invest Dermatol 46:584, 1966

25. Stumpf WE, Madhabananda S, Joshi SG: Oestrogen target cells in the skin. Experientia 30:196, 1974

26. Punnonen R: Effect of castration and peroral estrogen therapy on the skin. Acta Obstet Gynecol Scand 52:1, Suppl 21, 1972

27. Ferriman D: Human Hair Growth in Health and Disease. Springfield, Ill, Thomas, 1971

28. Hamilton JB, Mestler GE: Low values for sebum in eunuchs and oophorectomized women. Proc Soc Exp Biol Med 112:374, 1963

29. Silver AF, Montagna W, Karacan I: The effect of age on human eccrine sweating. In Montagna W (ed): Advances in Biology of Skin. Oxford, Pergamon, 1965

30. Marks R, Shahrad P: Aging and the effect of estrogens on the skin. In Beard RJ (ed): The Menopause. Lancaster, MTP Press, 1976, p 143

31. Kirk JE, Chieffi M: Variation with age in elasticity of skin and subcutaneous tissue in human individuals. J Gerontol 17:373, 1962

32. Hertz DG, Steiner JE, Zuckerman S, Pizanti S: Psychological and physical symptom formation in menopause. Psychother Psychosom 19:47, 1971

33. van Keep PA, Haspels AA: Oestrogen Therapy. Amsterdam, Exerpta Medica, 1977, p 21.

34. Utian WH: Clinical and metabolic effects of the menopause and the role of replacement oestrogen therapy. Unpublished Ph.D. Thesis, University of Cape Town, 1970

35. Milligan D, Drife JO, Short RV: Changes in breast volume during normal menstrual cycle and after oral contraceptives. Br Med J 4:494, 1975

36. Chan V, Besser GM, Landon J: Effects of oestrogen on urinary thyroxine secretion. Br Med J 4:699, 1972

5

Postmenopausal Osteoporosis

Van Keep mentions that he was asked long ago why grandmothers always have to be so small.[1] The possible answer, from an early classic paper on postmenopausal estrogen therapy,[2] was that postmenopausal women suffer progressive bone loss leading to osteoporosis, vertebral collapse, and loss of height. It was suggested that postmenopausal estrogen therapy would prevent this problem and the many related consequences.

Twenty-five years later the theory was still unconfirmed, leading to many statements of frustration such as that of Heaney in 1976: "In my opinion there have been few more glaring examples in recent years of a lack of scholarliness than in the controversy concerning estrogen therapy.... I feel that with a smaller investment of time and money than has to date been made, we could by now have had some clearer answers. However, we confront much the same uncertainty today that we started with."[3]

Fortunately, conscientious research is being done, and information is coming forth at an escalating pace. By mid-1977 the Endocrine Metabolic Advisory Committee and the Gynecology Advisory Committee of the United States Food and Drug Administration agreed that there was enough data to state that estrogens do prevent postmenopausal bone loss.[4] But there is still insufficient data to answer the most pertinent question of all. Can prevention of osteoporosis be maintained in the long term, and will this be reflected in a lower rate of bone fractures and their disabling consequences? The story behind the efforts at explaining osteoporosis and the attempts at its prevention is a fascinating one, and well deserves the following in-depth review.

DEFINITION

It was not until 1941 that Albright et al. described osteoporosis as a clinical entity.[5] Osteoporosis is a common clinical disorder which may cause backache or fracture in the elderly. It is notable for the reduced amount of bony tissue per unit volume of bone in the affected part or parts of the skeleton. Unlike osteomalacia, there are no known major and specific biochemical abnormalities in osteoporosis, and most authors agree that osteoporotic bone, while reduced in quantity, is essentially normal in chemical composition.[3,6]

Osteoporosis is defined as a bone disorder characterized by a progressive loss of bone mass until the skeleton is inadequate for mechanical support.[7] Trabecular bone loss is greater than cortical bone loss. For this reason, a stricter definition is sometimes applied, leaving the term osteoporosis for cases with crush fractures or when the percentage of bone, measured by acceptable parameters, falls below the lower normal limit associated with aging which is about 15 percent.[8] The normal loss of bone associated with aging can then be described by the term *osteopenia*. If further terminologic definition is required, then the excessive loss of cortical bone could be called "excessive osteopenia."[8] Both osteopenia and osteoporosis are generally considered to be disorders of calcium homeostasis.[3,8,9]

INCIDENCE AND CLINICAL SIGNIFICANCE

Well-defined prevalence, complication, and disability rates for osteoporosis are hard to come by. Nonetheless, the problem appears to be an enormous one, the extent of which became more obvious from about the mid-1950s onwards. It has become clear that a distinct relationship exists between osteoporosis and bone fractures. For example, of all patients with hip fracture, over 80 percent have preexisting osteoporosis.[10]

Stewart reported that femoral neck fractures occured three times more frequently in women than men,[11] and that such fractures were generally more common over the age of sixty. Confirmation quickly followed, as did evidence for a dramatic rise in lower forearm (Colles) fractures in women over the age of 40, which has no counterpart in men (Figure 5.1).[12-15] These forearm fractures, however, tend to occur some 10 to 15 years earlier than the femoral neck fractures,[11,13] suggesting that the association between menopause, osteoporosis, and an increased fracture rate may be partially influenced by other factors.[16-19]

Femoral Neck Fractures

Femoral neck fractures are common, and are a major cause of serious disability and death.[11,15,17] A regional survey from the United Kingdom confirms the extent of the problem, and suggests that it may even be increasing.[19] By the age of 90, 3 in every 100 women fractured their femoral neck per year. In this study the female preponderance of this injury was 3.17:1.[19] Of considerable import is the fact that in this particular study, one-fifth of patients admitted to hospital for femoral neck fractures died in hospital. The average length of hospital inpatient stay was over one month.[19] In the United States the only morbidity and mortality data reported were from the Commission on Professional and Hospital Activity. For 1972-73 they reported 135,000 hip fractures with over 10,000 deaths, over 80 percent of fractures and deaths in postmenopausal women. These figures were gathered from about one-third of all United States short-term hospitals.[17] Osteoporosis and hip fractures are predominantly the problem of whites, the condition being very rare in black populations.[18]

The potential cost to the patient and the community in terms of human suffering and financial burden is enormous. With an ever-increasing elderly population, the importance of prevention and effective treatment of femoral neck fractures speaks for itself. Otherwise, it can be expected that 1 percent of women living to age 70, and over 10 percent of those living beyond 85 will suffer a fracture of the hip, with the staggering morbidity and mortality described above.[11,19] It has been estimated that the annual cost of this single injury in Europe and North America in 1978 will exceed U.S. $2 billion.[20]

Lower Forearm Fractures

The relationship between sex, age, and the incidence of fractures of the lower forearm is apparent in Figure 5-1. Over 10 percent of women will fracture the lower forearm by age 70 and double that figure at age 85.[13-15] The incidence of wrist fractures eventually becomes 10 times higher than that of men. The mortality rates are not comparable to that of femoral neck fractures. The morbidity is difficult to define. Certainly, from an individual standpoint, such a fracture could make all the difference between self-dependence and the need for institutionalization.

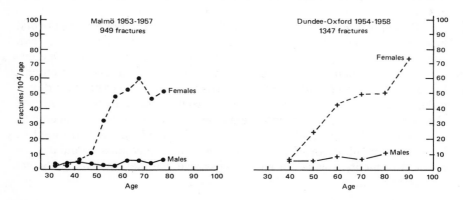

Figure 5-1.   Incidence of Colles fractures in relation to age, in Malmo[14] and Dundee-Oxford[15] (From Gallagher and Nordin: Front Horm Res 2:98, 1973. Courtesy of Karger Publishers).

Vertebral Crush Fractures

Data on the prevalence rates of vertebral crush fractures in the general population are inadequate. The symptomatic manifestation of vertebral crush fracture is acute or chronic back pain, and most statistics exist for this group. Even here there is room for statistical error, as trauma or weight bearing must be a factor in all fractures, and the unpredictability of this factor must account for some variability between the degree of bone loss and the presence of fractures.[21]

Despite these qualifications, 50 to 70 fractures are sustained per 1000 women per year after the menopause.[22] Up to 30 percent of healthy women in a Jewish home for the aged were found to have asymptomatic vertebral crush fractures.[23] It has also been shown that women attending hospital for backache have the same prevalence of osteoporosis as normal volunteer controls of similar age.[24] Statistics such as these have led Aitken to assume that "those women who are sufficiently motivated to attend hospital because of backache merely represent the tip of an iceberg of chronic musculo-skeletal malaise."[25]

METHODOLOGIC PROBLEMS IN BONE MEASUREMENT

There was, until fairly recently, a major problem in the investigation of the cause, development, and response to treatment of osteoporosis. This was the lack of a specific tool to actually establish the diagnosis of osteoporosis, and measure the change in bone density over any period of time.

Osteoporotic bone not only has less absolute volume than normal bone; morphologically it exhibits a greater loss of trabecular bone than cortical bone. Long bones are largely made up of cortical bone. Deeper, irregularly shaped bones invariably have a major trabecular element, but are difficult to get at for *in vivo* measurement. However, with developing osteoporosis there is some loss of cortical bone as well,[26] and the shafts of these long bones lend themselves more easily to measurement.

Some of the methods that have been evolved for measurement of bone density will be briefly listed and described. The most popular sites of measurement, because of easy access, are the metacarpals, proximal radius, and femur.

X-rays   Straight radiography of the spine or long bones is of little value in measuring bone density because of many obvious technologic problems including tube to film distance, exposure, soft tissue factors, film development, etc.

Bone Biopsy   Bone biopsy should be the ideal tool for studying bone. But it is often associated with unpleasant side effects, and its use as a technique for diagnosing simple osteoporosis can probably not be justified. Moreover, the interpretation of the material histologically is costly and time-consuming.

Trabecular Pattern Grading   The grading of the trabecular bone pattern at the proximal end of the femur known as the *Singh Index*,[27] is based on the bone structure rather than on the amount of bone in the proximal femur.[28] This index therefore represents the strength of the bone at the femoral neck. In practice it has less value when used to evaluate the vertebra.[29]

Radiogrammetry   One of the easiest methods for estimating bone mass relative to bone volume is the measurement on a straight radiograph of the cortical and total diameter of a long bone.[30] This *Barnett Nordin Index* proved to have a reproducibility error of greater than five percent, making it an insensitive index to assess long-term change in bone content.

Nordin and group have reduced this problem by converting the cortical/shaft into a cortical area/total area (CA/TA) ratio, derived as follows:

$$CA/TA = 1 - (1-C/T)^2$$

where C is cortical thickness and T is total diameter.[31]

X-ray Densitometry   Applied radiographic methods have been developed to measure the density of bones. More difficult than radiogrammetry, the techniques appear to offer better reproducibility.[25] These methods actually measure total bone density (cortical and trabecular bone plus bone marrow). Different bones will thus have individual characteristics.[25,32,33]

Metacarpal densitometry[33] is one method that has proved useful in practice.[25] An x-ray of the hand is taken combining an aluminum step wedge of known densities. The density of the aluminum standard and the midpoint of the third metacarpal is scanned and compared with a densitometer (Figure 5-2). The result is expressed in mm of aluminum giving the Aluminum Equivalent. If the metacarpal diameter at the scan site is corrected for, a Whole Bone Density is obtained as follows:

$$\frac{\text{Aluminum Equivalent}}{\text{metacarpal diameter in centimeters}} = \text{Whole Bone Density}^{33,34}$$

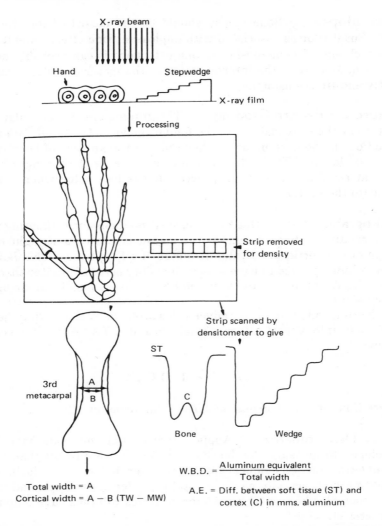

Figure 5-2. Diagrammatic representation of quantitative radiographic method of estimating bone mineral density. The results are expressed as whole bone density, the aluminum equivalent divided by the total width of the metacarpal (From Lindsay and Anderson, Radiography 44:21, 1978. Courtesy of Radiography).

Photon Absorptiometry   Another technique for measurement of bone mineral content *in vivo* is that of photon absorptiometry. The method is technically simple and noninvasive, involving a radioisotopic source (^{125}I or [241]Am) and a scintillation detector[35] (Figure 5-3). The site for measurement is placed between the two, and a direct mineral content computed from the amount of λ-radiation transfer that is blocked.

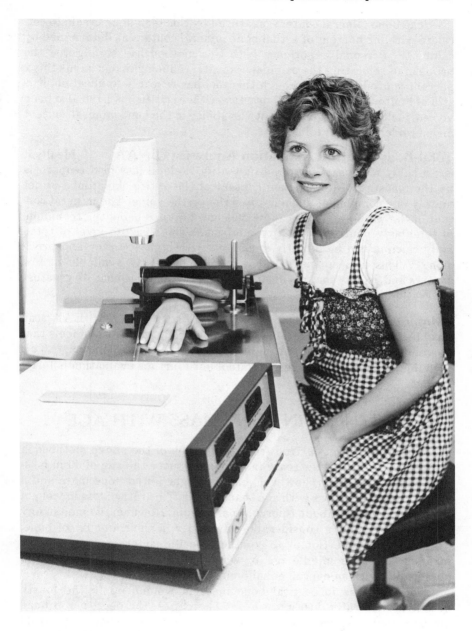

Figure 5–3. The instrumentation for measurement of bone density by photon absorptiometry. Note marker between fingers to enhance serial reproducibility by scanning the wrist at the same site. The digital computer readout is in front (Courtesy of Norland Instruments, Fort Atkinson, Wisconsin).

The bone mineral content measured by this technique is said to correlate within 2 percent of actual bone mineral content as determined by ashing.[36,37] Personal experience with this method has highlighted the problem of relocating the original scan site, reducing in our hands this 2 percent reproducibility. Though this tool has research application, it is still of limited value in clinical practice. Other criticisims have also been voiced, including a large inherent variability in the bone mineral content measurement of the radius.[38]

Total-Body Neutron Activation Analysis (TBNAA)   Ideally it is probably more satisfactory to quantify skeletal loss in osteoporosis by the measure of the calcium content of the entire skeleton, and not merely one component such as the wrist or the spine. The mineral content of the whole skeleton can be measured *in vivo* using the technique of total-body neutron activation analysis.[39] The absolute level of total-body calcium can be directly measured with high accuracy and precision.[38,39] This is a sophisticated technique presently available in few centers and, except for specific individual problems, still has its greatest application as a research tool.

Computed Axial Tomography (CAT scan)   The CAT scan has been applied to evaluation of cancellous bone, and Gordon feels that vertebral spongiosa can be well measured by utilizing this tool.[39A] This technique, too, remains a research tool until further evaluation is forthcoming.

CHANGES IN BONE MASS WITH AGE

The information derived from application of the above methods is as follows: There is a decrease in bone mass after the age of 40 in both men and women. Men, however, have a larger initial bone mass and a slower rate of bone loss with age than women. This rate of loss in women over 40 amounts to about 1 percent per annum. However, women in any age category show a considerable variability in their amount of bone. This raises the question as to whether specific factors are responsible for bone loss after middle age, or whether there is an individual bone personality with an overall equal bone gain and loss.[29]

The increase in cortical bone mass in women up to the fourth decade is illustrated in Figure 5-4.[29] Thereafter, the decrease in bone mass amounts to about 0.6 percent per year for the second metacarpal and 0.9 percent per year for the distal end of the radius. In all instances, this rate of loss appears to increase significantly during the sixth decade.[29,37] Ultimately, women will lose about a third of their bone mass, whereas men will only lose about 20 percent, and that at a much later age. This difference is well documented in Figure 5-5.

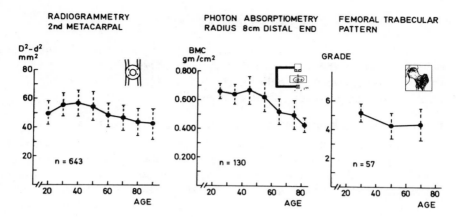

Figure 5–4.　Age pattern of bone changes in females measured by radio-grammetry at the second metacarpal, by photon absorptiometry at the distal end of the radius and by trabecular pattern grading at the upper end of the femur (From Dequeker et al.: Front Horm Res 3:116, 1975. Courtesy of Karger Publishers).

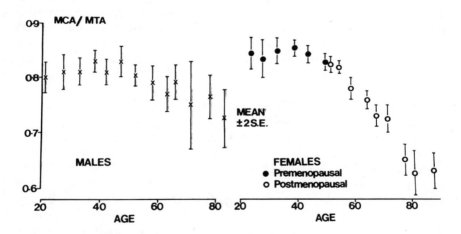

Figure 5–5.　Sex difference in bone loss with age as measured by the meta-carpal cortical area/total area ratio (Courtesy of Prof. BEC Nordin, MRC Mineral Metabolism Unit, Leeds, England).

ETIOLOGY OF OSTEOPOROSIS

Osteoporosis does not have a single etiology, and probably re-presents the end state of a condition with multiple causes, much as anemia has many possible causative factors.[3] Even individual cases may result from multiple factors working together.

Role of the Ovaries

Although Albright suggested as early as 1941 that diminished ovarian function and menopausal status were the major causative factors for osteoporosis,[5] it is only relatively recently that evidence for this relationship has been suitably documented.

BONE LOSS AFTER SPONTANEOUS MENOPAUSE   Ovarian agenesis was long ago reported to be complicated more frequently by osteoporosis.[40] Nordin et al. showed a specific relationship to exist between natural menopause and bone loss. They demonstrated a greater correlation between the time elapsed since natural menopause and parameters of bone mass, than between parameters of bone mass and chronological age.[6] When the indices of osteoporosis were related to the menopause, they observed decreases in vertebral density 5 years after menopause, decreased metacarpal cortical thickness about 10 years after menopause, and a reduction in femoral cortical thickness after about 15 years.[6]

There is also evidence to show a relationship between plasma hormone levels and osteoporosis. Marshall et al. reported a significant decrease in plasma androstenedione and estrone levels in women with osteoporosis compared to normal women. Women who had undergone oophorectomy had hormone concentrations intermediate between the normal and osteoporotic values.[41]

EFFECT OF OOPHORECTOMY IN PREMENOPAUSAL WOMEN   Retrospective studies had suggested that removal of normally functioning ovaries would result in a significant reduction in bone mineral.[42,43] Unfortunately, the controls used in these early studies were not well defined. A well-controlled investigation by Aitken and colleagues in Glasgow was also retrospective, but their groups were identical for all variables except one, namely the presence or absence of ovaries.[25,44] They reported that removal of functioning ovaries from women before the age of 45 was associated with premature bone loss, whereas oophorectomy after 45 had little if any additional effect on subsequent bone mineral loss.[44] They concluded that loss of ovarian function and loss of bone mineral were unlikely to be independent phenomena and that reduced ovarian function was probably the major determinant for loss of bone mineral with age.

These results are somewhat in conflict with a report by Gallagher et al. that removal of ovaries from premenopausal women of mean age 43.5 years is followed by significant calcium loss.[45] Utian's failure to find any significant change in the plasma calcium level with oophorectomy after age 45 would be more in agreement with Aitken's findings.[46] The discrepancy could be explained by reviewing data of Gallagher et al. which show their patient material to fall into both age groups, i.e., above and below 45 years. These studies taken overall appear to indicate that normally functioning ovaries exert a protective effect on the skeleton which is reduced and then lost during the perimenopause.[45]

POSSIBLE MECHANISM OF ACTION OF ESTROGENS ON BONE
Osteoporosis can be called a "disease of theories" when it comes to explaining the precise relationship between ovarian function and bone metabolism. The answer is not known. Many possible mechanisms have been considered of which the following are possibilities.

Anticatabolic Effect on Collagenous Tissues
Estrogens may have an anticatabolic effect on collagenous tissues in general. Hydroxyproline is an amino acid present almost exclusively in collagen. Nordin et al. reported an increase in hydroxyproline excretion after menopause which they attributed to a rise in bone resorption.[8] However, Aloia et al. demonstrated that hydroxyproline excretion in postmenopausal and osteoporotic women was not related to either regional or total bone mass, suggesting that the major determinant of bone mass in later life is the amount of bone placed in the skeletal bank during the phase of skeletal growth.[47] Their data thus failed to provide any evidence that there is a difference in bone turnover between osteoporotic women and younger postmenopausal women, or that osteoporosis arises from a sub-population of women with rapid bone loss. This study lacked premenopausal controls and both groups studied were of different ages.[47]

Altered Sensitivity of Bone to Parathyroid Hormones
Bone may be unduly sensitive to the action of parathyroid hormones in the absence of estrogen. It will be recalled that the function of parathyroid hormones (PTH) is to maintain a normal plasma calcium. It achieves this through resorption of calcium from bone. There is also an increase in renal tubular resorption of calcium and probably an increased intestinal absorption of calcium. PTH inhibits renal tubular reabsorption of phosphate. There is no evidence for a specific inhibition of parathyroid hormone by estrogens, although circumstantial evidence for a nonspecific effect does exist.[8] For example, estrogens have a hypocalcemic action in postmenopausal and oophorectomized women.[45,46] Estrogen administration to postmenopausal hyperparathyroid patients has also been shown to reduce calcium loss[47A] and hydroxyproline.[47] Indeed the incidence of primary hyperparathyroidism is lower in premenopausal women. One explanation for this is that estrogens may have the ability to mask the disease.[47]

Estrogens have been demonstrated *in vitro* to inhibit the calcium mobilizing effect of parathyroid hormone.[48] The *in vivo* effect of estrogen on parathyroid hormone activity still remains to be proven.

Effect on Calcitonin   Estrogens may exert their effect via calcitonin, either by increasing tissue response to calcitonin or by actually increasing calcitonin secretion, but as yet this idea remains conjectural.[25] Certainly, a menstrual cyclicity in calcium regulating hormone has been reported,[49] and estrogen treatment of castrated rats increases the level of measurable calcitonin.[50]

Inhibitory Action on Osteoclastic Function   Frost was the first to suggest that postmenopausal osteoporosis is a disorder of osteoclastic activity, but he could not explain the cause for an increase in such activity.[51] Estrogen does appear to reduce the number of bone resorbing surfaces seen on iliac crest biopsy.[52]

Role of Calcium Deficiency

Present information is compatible with the concept that estrogen deficiency is one of two main factors in the genesis of postmenopausal osteoporosis, the other being malabsorption of calcium.[31,41,53] Calcium absorption is generally reduced in spinal osteoporosis and this malabsorption of calcium can be corrected with large doses of vitamin D.[54,55]

Calcium absorption is generally completed three to five hours after an average meal.[56] Thus no calcium is being absorbed during the night, and calcium lost in the urine between midnight and breakfast probably represents a loss via skeletal resorption. If there is sufficient bone formation during the day to balance the loss at night, then the skeletal mass should remain in balance. Skeletal turnover, however, is slow, although presumably sufficient in young people to maintain the status quo.

A menstrual cyclicity has been shown to exist in calcium-regulating hormones.[49] The timing of this suggests an estrogen effect, lending support to the theory that estrogen inhibits parathyroid hormone-induced bone resorption. Loss of estrogenic activity would help explain the higher early morning urine calcium of women.

Inevitably, osteoporosis would appear to result from an impaired adaptation to calcium deficiency. As calcium absorption falls with age, parathyroid hormone is activated, and bone resorption and calcium loss increased. Animal experimentation would support the theory that calcium deficiency and estrogen are additive factors in the genesis of osteoporosis. Oophorectomy and calcium deficiency each reduce bone mass in the adult rat, but the greatest effect is seen when they are combined.[57]

Miscellaneous Factors

PREGNANCY AND LACTATION   Pregnancy and lactation are both associated with considerable calcium turnover. Little is known about the effect of these events on bone mass, although such information would be of considerable potential value.

SMOKING   Daniell has warned against smoking in the slender menopausal patient, suggesting that this individual is apparently at severe risk for osteoporosis.[58] This theory is still in need of confirmation.

EXERCISE   It is extremely likely that exercise may prevent or reduce involutional bone loss. Total body calcium has been shown to increase with exercise over a time span of one year, but long-term studies of specific bone parameters are necessary.[58A]

DIFFERENTIAL DIAGNOSIS OF OSTEOPOROSIS

Postmenopausal osteoporosis is often termed "primary osteoporosis" and accounts for some 95 percent of total cases of osteoporosis. Bone loss can also occur as a problem secondary to diseases such as rheumatoid arthritis[25] or to drug therapies. Such possible causative factors for secondary osteoporosis are listed below.

1. Immobilization and weightlessness
2. Drugs
   a. Corticosteroids
   b. Cytotoxic agent
   c. Heparin
3. Endocrine
   a. Hyperthyroidism
   b. Primary hyperparathyroidism
   c. Hyperadrenalism (Cushing's syndrome)
4. Dietary and malabsorption
   a. Calcium deficiency
   b. Intestinal malabsorption syndrome
   c. Upper gastrointestinal tract surgery
   d. Vitamin C deficiency (scurvy)
   e. Alcoholism
5. Chronic renal failure
6. Vitamin D deficiency
7. Rheumatoid arthritis
8. Hereditary — osteogenesis imperfecta

Detailed discussion of these problems is beyond the scope of this monograph. Nonetheless, the above factors should be considered in the clinical workup of osteoporosis. These problems can usually be excluded on the history, physical examination, and routine screening tests, which should include plasma measurements of calcium, phosphorous, alkaline phosphatase, and complete blood count.[25] If in doubt, thyroid and renal studies may be necessary.

OSSEOUS EFFECTS OF EXOGENOUS SEX HORMONE THERAPY

There are numerous papers in the literature acclaiming estrogen as a cure for osteoporosis. Close scrutiny of most of these papers invariably exposes fundamental problems in the methodology, including case selection, lack of randomization, failure to evaluate prospectively, inappropriate measures of bone response, etc. In essence the problem has necessitated an evaluation of several levels of effect of therapy, some of which have been successfully performed and others still awaiting conclusive evidence. These levels, which will be discussed individually, are as follows:

1. The effect of sex hormone treatment on calcium balance.
2. The effect of such treatment on bone density; that is, is postmenopausal bone loss preventable?
3. The effect of hormonal therapy on bone fracture rates.
4. The use of these hormones for treatment of established osteoporosis. Is postmenopausal bone loss reversible?

Induction of Positive Calcium Balance   Several investigators have demonstrated exogenous estrogen therapy to be extremely effective in reducing plasma calcium and inorganic phosphorous values in oophorectomized women[59,60,61] (Figure 5-6), that is, to reverse the rise in plasma and urinary calcium and phosphorous values that generally follows menopause and castration.[45,62,63] The effect of this response is to create a positive calcium balance.[45] The reason for this response is presumably the inhibition of bone resorption.[64]

Different estrogens appear to vary in their ability to reduce plasma calcium values.[46,65] The variability in effect could be explained by different dose-responses, and Utian has proposed the measurement of the fasting plasma calcium response to estrogen treatment as a specific test of estrogen potency.[59]

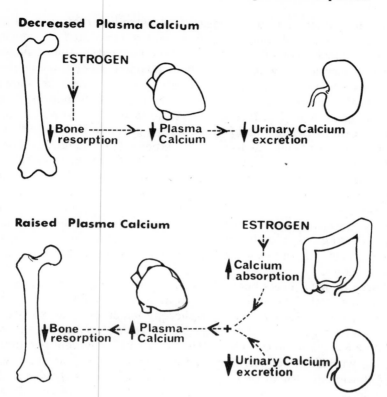

Figure 5-6. Two theoretical levels of effect of estrogen on plasma calcium. In practice estrogen administration is reflected in decreased plasma calcium levels and urinary calcium excretion (upper diagram), and not by elevated plasma calcium, shown in the alternate model (lower diagram). The effect of estrogen on plasma calcium, therefore, confirms the level of action to be at the bone itself (From Utian: S Afr Med J 49:433, 1975. Courtesy South African Medical Journal).

Prevention of Bone Loss   There is now more than sufficient evidence to make a definitive statement that estrogens prevent bone loss. However, some qualifications are necessary.

The earliest studies of estrogen on bone loss suggested that such therapy would prevent the normally expected loss in height shown to occur in postmenopausal women.[2,66] These studies could be criticized for failure of randomization and inadequacy or lack of suitable controls.

Prospective controlled studies have confirmed the protective effect of estrogen against bone loss. One of the best prospective trials has been reported by Aitken et al. from Glasgow.[25,67] Estrogen treatment started within two months of bilateral oophorectomy prevented subsequent bone mineral loss. In quantitative terms, placebo-treated women showed a profound decrease in bone mass of about 4.5 percent per annum during the first two years of observation. The estrogen-treated women showed a change of less than 0.2 percent per annum.[25,67] Confirmation of this study has come from Nordin's group at the MRC Mineral Metabolism Research Unit at Leeds,[68] and from Heaney's group in Nebraska,[64] both demonstrating estrogens to prevent the expected postmenopausal bone loss (Figure 5-7). Moreover, Lindsay et al. have shown this skeletal protective effect to last as long as eight years.[69] They believe estrogen therapy to be effective in preventing bone loss when prescribed at any age after menopause.[70] They have reported a similar effect for progestogen therapy as well.[71] Further recent reports for an estrogen protective effect against bone loss are the ten-year double-blind prospective study of Nachtigall and co-workers,[71A] and a three-year study by Dalen and co-workers.[71B]

Three major aspects need emphasis. First, estrogen does not prevent all age-related bone loss. It does appear to abolish the sex difference, however. Second, estrogen therapy needs to be administered over a prolonged period of time to be effective. Lindsay et al. have shown the bone mineral content to fall at a rate of 2.5 percent per annum following withdrawal of estrogen. Patients treated for four years who were followed up without therapy for the next four years showed no difference in bone measurements over patients who had received placebo for a full eight years (Figure 5-8). Thirdly, therapy may be more effective when administered within three years of the menopause.[71A] Before

Potential Prevention of Bone Fractures

There is very little documentation for an effect of estrogens in protecting against osteoporotic fractures. In theory, this would be expected; in practice, the matter must be considered unproven. Ideally, a large-scale, randomized, prospective, double-blind trial is required. Logistically and practically this is extremely difficult to accomplish. An alternate possibility is to await the effect of current therapeutic practices to be reflected on epidemiologic statistics for fracture rates, much as the initial evidence was suggested for a relationship between estrogen usage and uterine cancer. This, of course, would be less satisfactory than direct evidence.

Some early evidence has begun to appear. For example, Gordan et al. have described almost complete cessation of fracture in patients after starting estrogens.[72] Burch et al. in a prospective study of 11,026 patient years of estrogen therapy in hysterectomized women, noted a decrease in the incidence of wrist fractures and a total absence of hip fractures.[73] Hammond and co-workers also reported a lower rate of development of

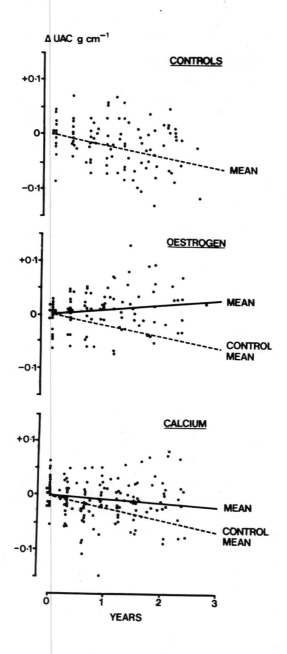

Figure 5–7.   Sequential changes in mineral content of ulna in postmenopausal women observed at four-to-six month intervals over two years or
more. Women in the untreated control group continued to lose bone during
the two years, whereas the estrogen group lost none. Loss in the calcium-
treated group was intermediate (From Horsman et al.: Br Med J 2:789, 1977.
Courtesy of Professor BEC Nordin and the Publishers).

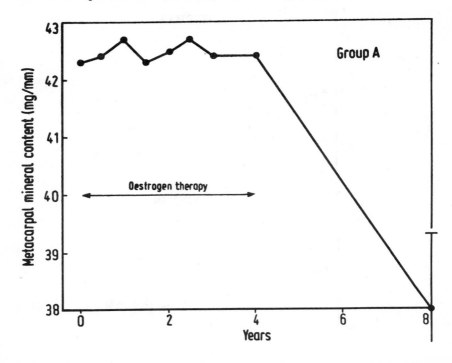

Figure 5–8.   Effects of withdrawal of estrogen therapy on bone mineral content after 4 years of active treatment (From Lindsay et al.: Lancet 1:1325 1978. Courtesy of Dr. R. Lindsay and Lancet).

osteoporosis and fractures in estrogen-treated patients, but the study was retrospective and inadequately controlled and defined.[73A] Specific deficiencies exist in each of the above studies, but the promise of a preventive against osteoporotic fractures is likely to be proven.

Treatment of Established Osteoporosis   Until recently it was believed that sex hormone therapy did not result in new bone formation.[3,7] New evidence suggests that during the early years of therapy there may be an actual increase in bone density.[71A,74] These results have been confirmed in a study suggesting estrogen to stimulate subperiosteal bone apposition.[68]

Current opinion is that sex hormones can be given to patients once they develop osteoporosis. A palliative effect can be expected in that further skeletal loss may be halted.[64] However, for all practical purposes it is unlikely that estrogen therapy alone will be successful in restoring bone mass to any major degree.

OTHER POSSIBLE THERAPEUTIC AGENTS

Several other therapeutic agents have been described for the prevention of bone loss or even for potentially increasing skeletal volume. The following is a brief list of the more promising ones.

Calcium   Postmenopausal bone loss can be delayed by calcium supplements.[64,68] This effect is weaker than that of estrogen used alone (Figure 5-7).[64,68] The dosage of oral calcium required is high, Recker et al. giving 2600 mg of calcium carbonate daily,[64] equivalent to 1.04g of elemental calcium per day. Through personal experiences, patients on such high dosage tend to suffer nausea.

The theoretical explanation for the effectiveness of calcium in preventing bone loss has been postulated by Heaney.[75] Sex hormones may "set" the level of bone sensitivity to parathyroid hormone (PTH). Natural or surgical menopause increases bone sensitivity to PTH but does not change the sensitivity of its other target organs, the gut and kidney. Calcium homeostasis can only be maintained by increased resorption from bone. Calcium supplementation provides amounts necessary for the homeostasis and thus the decrease in bone resorption can be accounted for.[68,75] Calcium loss is maximal during the night. A late evening supplement of calcium has been proven effective in reducing this loss and the suggestion has been made that such therapy is therefore best administered as a single late-evening dose rather than in divided doses throughout the day.[76]

Vitamin D and Analogues   The fact that older women absorb calcuim less effectively[21,77] has provided the rationale for giving vitamin D and its analogues. Large, unphysiologic doses of vitamin D were required in order to achieve an effect.[77]

Developing research at the MRC Mineral Metabolism Unit at Leeds has shown that 1 α-hydroxy-vitamin D_3 (1 α-OHD$_3$), a synthetic vitamin D analogue which is hydroxylated by the liver into an active metabolite called 1,25-dihydroxyvitamin D_3 (1,25 α-(OH)$_2$D$_3$), is effective in raising calcium absorption in doses as small as 1 or 2 μg per day. A side effect was hypercalcemia with loss of much of the extra absorbed calcium in the urine. The most recent evidence suggests that a positive calcium balance can only be induced if estrogens are administered in combination with 1 α-OHD$_3$. Moreover, calcium supplementation is also recommended in patients with low dietary intakes of calcium.[78]

Fluoride   Studies of bone biopsy specimens in patients on fluoride treatment have shown stimulation of production of osteoblasts.[79] Unfortunately, the newly formed osteoid tissue is poorly mineralized, resulting in the development of secondary hyperparathyroidism and a histological picture of osteomalacia.[80] It is possible that combined therapy with sodium fluoride, vitamin D, and calcium may avoid this problem.[81] Further experience is awaited at this point and this form of therapy is not generally favored.

Calcitonin   Early evidence suggests that low dose porcine calcitonin treatment decreases bone resorption and urinary calcium excretion, and increases bone accretion in postmenopausal osteoporotic women.[82] The predominant result seems to be hypocalcemia, however. Jowsey et al. have attempted to give calcium and salmon calcitonin, but this did not result in change of bone mass. She therefore stated that it seems unlikely that calcitonin has any additional desirable effect in the disease.[83]

Growth Hormone and Parathyroid Hormone   Both growth hormone[84] and human synthetic parathyroid hormone fragment (hPTH)[85] appreciably increase bone turnover with little change in calcium balance. The latter does have an osteoclastic effect and further basic research is necessary before these agents can be introduced clinically.

CONCLUSION

Osteoporosis is a significant problem in white women after menopause. It is associated with a high rate of bone fracture and subsequent morbidity and mortality. With an ever-increasing elderly population the extent of this problem will escalate unless determined efforts are made to prevent its development in susceptible individuals.

Despite a considerable amount of disagreement on the mechanism of effect of ovarian hormones on bone metabolism, a general consensus does exist for actual recognition of postmenopausal osteoporosis as a real entity. Spontaneous ovarian failure with natural menopause and premature ovarian failure by castration both result in detectable loss of bone. Bone loss is particularly accelerated if ovaries are removed before the age of 45. Conversely, until the age of 45 the ovary appears to have a protective effect on the skeleton. These findings have been confirmed by bone density and chemical studies, and a relationship between hormone levels and osteoporosis has also been reported. After the age of 45 years this protective effect is progressively lost.

There have been two fundamentally different approaches to treatment of the problem: prevention and restoration. One significant approach to prevention is avoidance of premature menopause. The most frequent cause for this problem is removal of normally functioning ovaries from women undergoing hysterectomy for benign causes. A strong case can be made for conservation of such ovaries (Chapter 10).

Another approach to prevention is directed at reducing bone resorption so that bone formation can keep in step. Here, the use of hormones, calcium supplements, and vitamin D and its analogues has been clearly shown to be of value in delaying and probably preventing bone loss. What is yet to be satisfactorily proven is the effect of this approach in the long term on bone fracture rates and the related morbidity and mortality statistics.

The attempted restoration of skeletal mass after a decline has already occurred is the alternative approach to the problem of osteoporosis. This would require the ability of a therapeutic agent to stimulate new bone formation. Fluoride, human synthetic parathyroid hormone fragment (hPTH), and growth hormone, with or without vitamin D and calcium supplements, have shown some ability to stimulate new osteoblastic activity. For all practical purposes, however, no treatment has yet been proven to be safe, practical, and effective in promoting substantial new normal bone formation.

It can therefore be concluded that bone metabolism, and more specifically bone loss, does have a relationship to declining ovarian activity. Bone loss can be prevented by not removing functional ovaries unnecessarily or by administering specific supplemental therapy over a prolonged period of time to appropriately selected females at risk. The problem in this respect is to select the at-risk population who should be offered treatment on a long-term basis. At this point in time that population has not been adequately defined, despite research directed at this problem, and patients are selected for therapy on a relatively empirical basis.

References

1.   van Keep PA, Haspels AA: Oestrogen Therapy. Amsterdam, Excerpta Medica, 1977

2.   Wallach S, Henneman PH: Prolonged estrogen therapy in postmenopausal women. JAMA 171:1637, 1959

3.   Heaney RP: Estrogens and postmenopausal osteoporosis. Clin Obstet Gynecol 19:791, 1976

4.   Gordan GS, Genant HK: Postmenopausal osteoporosis is a preventable disease. Contemp Obstet Gynecol 11:47, 1978

5.   Albright F, Smith PH, Richardson AM: Postmenopausal osteoporosis, its clinical features. JAMA 116:2465, 1941

6.   Nordin BEC, MacGregor J, Smith DA: The incidence of osteoporosis in normal women: its relation to age and the menopause. Q J Med 35:25, 1966

7.   Utian WH: Oestrogens and osteoporosis. S Afr Med J 45:879, 1971

8.   Nordin BEC, Gallagher SC, Aaron JE, Horsman A: Post-menopausal osteopenia and osteoporosis. Front Horm Res 3:131, 1975

9.   Heaney RP: A Unified Concept of Osteoporosis. A Second Look in Osteoporosis. New York, Grune and Stratton, 1970

10.   Stevens J, Freedman DA, Nordin BEC, Barnett E: The incidence of osteoporosis in patients with femoral neck fracture. J Bone Joint Surg 44:520, 1962

11.   Stewart IM: Fractures of neck of femur. Incidence and implications. Br Med J 1:698, 1955

12.   Buhr AJ, Cooke AM: Fracture patterns. Lancet 1:531, 1959

13.   Bauer GCH: Epidemiology of fracture in aged persons. A preliminary investigation in fracture etiology. Clin Orthop 17:219, 1960

14.   Alffram PA: An epidemiologic study of cervical and trochanteric fractures of the femur in an urban population. Acta Orthop Scand Suppl 65: 1964

15.   Knowelden J, Buhr AJ, Dunbar O: Incidence of fractures in persons over 35 years of age. A report to the MRC working party on fractures in the elderly. Br J Prev Soc Med 18:130, 1964

16.   Newton-John HP, Morgan DB: Osteoporosis, disease or senescence? Lancet 1:232, 1968

17.   Commission on Professional and Hospital Activities: Hospital Mortality, PAS Hospitals, United States 1972-1973, Ann Arbor, 1975

18.   Gyepes M, Mellins HZ, Katz I: The low incidence of fracture of the hip in the Negro. JAMA 181:133, 1962

19.   Gallannaugh SC, Martin A, Millard PH: Regional survey of femoral neck fractures. Br Med J 2:1496, 1976

20.   Editorial: Treatment of osteoporosis. Br Med J 1:1303, 1978

21.   Gallagher JC, Aaron J, Horsman A, et al.: The crush fracture syndrome in postmenopausal women. J Clin Endocrinol Metab 2:293, 1973

22.   Iskrant AP, Smith RW: Osteoporosis in women 45 years and over related to subsequent fractures. Public Health Rep 84:33, 1969

23.   Gershon-Cohen J, Rechtman AM, Schraer H, Blumberg N: Asymptomatic fractures in osteoporotic spines of the aged. JAMA 153:625, 1953

24.   Smith DA, Anderson JB, Shimmins J, Speirs CF, Barnett E: Mineral and density changes in bone with age in normal and pathological states. In: Progress in Methods of Bone Mineral Measurement. Washington, DC, N.I.H., U.S. Dept of Health, Education, Welfare 1968, p 177

25.   Aitken JM: Bone metabolism in post-menopausal women. In Beard R (ed): The Menopause. Lancaster, MTP Press, 1976, p 95

26.   Aitken JM, Smith CB, Horton PW, et al.: The interrelationships between bone mineral at different skeletal sites in male and female cadaver. J Bone Joint Surg 56B:370, 1974

27.   Singh M, Magrath AR, Maini PS: Changes in trabecular pattern of the upper end of the femur as an index of osteoporosis. J Bone Joint Surg 52:457, 1970

28.   Kranendonk DH, Jurist JM, Gun Lee H: Femoral trabecular patterns and bone mineral content. J Bone Joint Surg 54:1472, 1972

29.   Dequeker J, Burssens A, Creytens G, Bouillon R: Aging of bone: its relation to osteoporosis and osteoarthrosis in postmenopausal women. Front Horm Res 3:116, 1975

30.   Barnett E, Nordin BEC: The radiologic diagnosis of osteoporosis. Clin Radiol 11:166, 1960

31.   Gallagher JC, Nordin BEC: Oestrogens and calcium metabolism. Front Horm Res 2:98, 1973

32.   Nordin BEC, Barnett E, MacGregor J, Nisbet J: Lumbar spine densitometry. Br Med J 1:1793, 1962

33.   Anderson JB, Shimmins J, Smith DA: A new technique for the measurement of metacarpal density. Br J Radiol 39:443, 1966

34.   Lindsay R, Anderson JB: Radiological determination of changes in bone mineral content. Radiography 44:21, 1978

35.   Cameron JR, Sorenson J: Measurement of bone mineral in vivo: an improved method. Science 142:5, 1963

36.   Cameron JR, Mazess RB, Sorenson JA: Precision and accuracy of bone mineral determination by direct photon absorptiometry. Invest Radiol 3:141, 1968

37.   Boyd RM, Cameron EC, McIntosh HW, Walker UR: Measurement of bone mineral content in vivo using photon absorptiometry. Can Med Assoc J 111:1201, 1974

38.   Cohn SH, Ellis KJ, Wallach S, et al.: Absolute and relative deficit in total-skeletal calcium and radial bone mineral in osteoporosis. J Nucl Med 15:428, 1974

39.   Cohn SH, Dombrowski CS: Measurement of total body calcium, sodium, chlorine, nitrogen and phosphorus in man by in vivo neutron activation analysis. J Nucl Med 12:499, 1971

39A.   Utian WH, Gordon GS: Metabolic changes due to menopause and their response to oestrogen. In van Keep PA, Serr DM, Greenblatt R (eds): Female and Male Climacteric, Lancaster, MTP Press, 1979, p 89

40.   Turner HH: Syndrome of infantilism, congenital webbed neck and cubitus valgus. Endocrinology 23:566, 1938

41.   Marshall DH, Crilly RG, Nordin BEC: Plasma androstenedione and oestrone levels in normal and osteoporotic postmenopausal women. Br Med J 2:1177, 1977

42.   Meema HE, Bunker ML, Meema S: Loss of compact bone due to menopause. Obstet Gynecol 26:333, 1965

43.   Nordin BEC, Young MM, Bentley B, Ormondroyd P, Sykes J: Lumbar spine densitometry methodology and results in relation to the menopause. Clin Radiol 19:459, 1968

44.   Aitken JM, Hart DM, Anderson JB, et al: Osteoporosis after oophorectomy for non-malignant disease in premenopausal women. Br Med J 2:325, 1973

45.   Gallagher JC, Young MM, Nordin BEC: Effects of artificial menopause on plasma and urine calcium and phosphate. Clin Endocrinol 1:57, 1972

46.   Utian WH: Effects of oophorectomy and subsequent oestrogen therapy on plasma calcium and phosphorus. S Afr J Obstet Gynecol 10:8, 1972

47.   Aloia JF, Cohn SH, Zanzi I, Abesamis C, Ellis K: Hydroxyproline peptides and bone mass in postmenopausal and osteoporotic women. J Clin Endocrinol Metab 47:314, 1978

47A.   Gallagher JC, Nordin BEC: Treatment with oestrogens of primary hyper-parathyroidism in postmenopausal women. Lancet 1:503, 1972

48.   Atkins D, Zanelli JM, Peacock M, Nordin BEC: The effect of oestrogens on the response of bone to parathyroid hormone in vitro. J Endocrinol 54:107, 1972

49.   Pitkin RM, Reynolds WA, Williams GA, Hargis GK: Calcium regulating hormones during the menstrual cycle. J Clin Endocrinol Metab 47:626, 1978

50.   Klotz HP, Delorme ML, Ochoa R, Aussenard C: Hormones sexuelles et secretion de calcitonine. Sem Hop Paris 51:1333, 1975

51.   Frost HM: Postmenopausal osteoporosis: a disturbance in osteoclasia. J Am Geriatr Soc 9:1078, 1961

52.   Riggs BL, Jowsey J, Goldsmith RS, et al: Short- and long-term effects of estrogen and synthetic anabolic hormone in postmenopausal osteoporosis. J Clin Invest 51:1659, 1972

53.   Gallagher JC, Riggs L, Eisman J, Arnaud S, Deluca H: Impaired intestinal calcium absorption in postmenopausal osteoporosis. Clin Res 24:360A, 1976

54.   Marshall DH, Nordin BEC: The effect of 1 α-hydroxyvitamin D_3 with and without oestrogens on calcium balance in post-menopausal women. Clin Endocrinol 7:159S, 1977

55.   Marshall DH, Gallagher JC, Guha P, et al.: The effect of 1 α hydroxy-cholecalciferol and hormone therapy on the calcium balance of post-menopausal osteoporosis. Calcif Tissue Res (Suppl) 22:78, 1977

56.   Birge SJ, Peck WA, Berman M, Whedon GD: Study of calcium absorption in man: a kinetic analysis and physiologic model. J Clin Invest 48:1705, 1969

57.   Hodgkinson A, Aaron JE, Horsman A, McLachlan MSF, Nordin BEC: Effect of oophorectomy and calcium deprivation on bone mass in the rat. Clin Sci Mol Med 54:439, 1978

58.   Daniell HW: Osteoporosis of the slender smoker. Arch Int Med 136:298, 1976

58A.   Aloia JF, Cohn SH, Ostuni JA, et al: Prevention of involutional bone loss by exercise. Ann Intern Med 89:356, 1978

59.   Utian WH: Osteoporosis, oestrogens and oophorectomy: A proposed new test of oestrogenic potency. S Afr Med J 49:433, 1975

60.   Jasani C, Nordin BEC, Smith DA, Swanson I: Spinal osteoporosis and the menopause. Proc R Soc Med 58:441, 1965

61.   Young MM, Jasani C, Smith DA, Nordin BEC: Some effects of ethinyl oestradiol on calcium and phosphorus metabolism in osteoporosis. Clin Sci 34:411, 1968

62.   Young MM, Nordin BEC: Calcium metabolism and the menopause. Proc R Soc Med 60:1137, 1967

63.   Szymendera J, Madajewicz S: Calcium metabolism after castration. Lancet 2:1091, 1967

64.   Recker RR, Saville PD, Heaney RP: Effect of estrogens and calcium carbonate on bone loss in postmenopausal women. Ann Intern Med 87:649, 1977

65.   Utian WH: Comparative trial of P 1496, a new non-steroidal oestrogen analogue. Br Med J 1:579, 1973

66.   Hernberg CA: Treatment of postmenopausal osteoporosis with estrogens and androgens. Acta Endocrinol 34:51, 1960

67.   Aitken JM, Hart DM, Lindsay R: Oestrogen replacement therapy for prevention of osteoporosis after oophorectomy. Br Med J 3:515, 1973

68.   Horsman A, Gallagher JC, Simpson M, Nordin BEC: Prospective trial of oestrogen and calcium in postmenopausal women. Br Med J 2:789, 1977

69.   Lindsay R, Hart DM, Maclean A, et al.: Bone response to termination of oestrogen treatment. Lancet 1:1325, 1978

70.   Lindsay R, Hart DM: Effect of oestrogens on postmenopausal bone loss. Br Med J 2:1087, 1977

71.   Lindsay R, Hart DM, Purdie D, et al.: Comparative effects of oestrogen and a progestogen on bone loss in postmenopausal women. Clin Sci Mol Med 54:193, 1978

71A.   Nachtigall LE, Nachtigall RH, Nachtigall RD, Beckman EM: Estrogen replacement therapy I: A 10-year prospective study in the relationship to osteoporosis. Obstet Gynecol 53:277, 1979

71B.   Dalen N, Furuhjelm M, Jacobson B, Lamke B: Changes in bone mineral content in women with natural menopause during treatment with female sex hormones. Acta Obstet Gynecol Scand 57:435, 1978

72.   Gordan GS, Picchi J, Roof BS: Antifracture efficacy of long-term estrogens for osteoporosis. Trans Assoc Am Physicians 86:326, 1973

73.   Burch JC, Byrd BF, Vaughn WK: The effects of long-term estrogen administration to women following hysterectomy. Front Horm Res 3:208, 1975

73A.   Hammond CB, Jelovsek FR, Lee KL, et al.: Effects of long-term estrogen replacement therapy. I Metabolic effects. Am J Obstet Gynecol 133:525, 1979

74.   Lindsay R., Hart DM, Aitken JM, et al.: Long-term prevention of postmenopausal osteoporosis by oestrogen. Evidence for an increased bone mass after delayed onset of oestrogen treatment. Lancet 1:1038, 1976

75.   Heaney RP: A unified concept of osteoporosis. Am J Med 39:877, 1965

76.   Belchetz PE, Lloyd MW, Johns RGS, Cohen RD: Effect of late night calcium supplements on overnight urinary calcium excretion in premenopausal and postmenopausal women. Br Med J 2:510, 1973

77.   Nordin BEC, Wilkinson R, Marshall DH, et al.: Calcium absorption in the elderly. In Neilsé SP, Hjorting-Hance E (eds): Calcified Tissues. Copenhagen, FADL Publishing, 1976, p 42

78.   Marshall DH, Nordin BEC: The effect of 1 α-hydroxyvitamin D_3 with and without oestrogens on calcium balance in post-menopausal women. Clin Endocrinol 7 (Suppl): 159S, 1977

79.   Jowsey J, Schenk RK, Reutter FW: Some results of the effect of fluoride on bone tissue in osteoporosis. J Clin Endocrinol 28:869, 1968

80.   Bernstein D, Cohen P: Use of sodium fluoride in the treatment of osteoporosis. J Clin Endocrinol 27:197, 1967

81.   Jowsey J, Riggs BL, Kelly PJ, Hoffman DL: Effect of combined therapy with sodium fluoride, vitamin D and calcium in osteoporosis. Am J Med 53:43, 1972

82.   Milhaud G, Talbot JN, Coutris G: Calcitonin treatment of postmenopausal osteoporosis. Evaluation of efficacy by principal components analysis. Biomedicine 23:223, 1975

83.   Jowsey J, Riggs BL, Kelly PJ, Hoffman DL: Calcium and salmon calcitonin in treatment of osteoporosis. J Clin Endocrinol Metab 47:633, 1978

84.   Haas HG, Dambacher MA, Goschke H, et al.: Growth hormone in osteoporosis. Calcif Tissue Res 21, Suppl 467, 1976

85.   Reeve J, Tregear GW, Parsons JA: Preliminary trial of low doses of human parathyroid hormone 1-34 peptide in treatment of osteoporosis. Calcif Tissue Res 21, Suppl 469, 1976

6
Cardiovascular and Blood Lipid Changes

Recent serious concern about coronary heart disease (CHD) is a result of its spectacular increase during this century to become one of the leading causes of death in developed countries. Almost a quarter of all deaths in men and 13 percent in women are now due to CHD. This sex-related difference in incidence of CHD stimulated questions as to the cause of the problem. Inevitably, premature hopes for prevention of CHD were also raised.

Both normal climacteric and castration appear to be related to alterations in lipid metabolism, the development of atherosclerotic vascular disease, and the incidence of CHD. There is no uniform agreement about the subject, and at best the relationship appears to be indirect. Moreover, the initial optimism that estrogen replacement therapy would prevent CHD was followed by an about turn, suggesting that these hormones could of themselves be risk factors for the development of CHD.

These conflicting ideas have generated intensive research, the results of which have begun to appear. As in all too many areas of science, the problem is more complex than originally anticipated; for example, different estrogens inducing different plasma lipid responses. Nonetheless, some clarification is possible.

CORONARY RISK FACTORS

Atherosclerosis is a metabolic disease that is influenced by many factors. It is characterized by deposition of lipid in the arterial wall, a disease process leading to narrowing of coronary arteries and eventually coronary thrombosis, ischemia, and myocardial infarction.[1-3] *Arteriosclerosis* is a general term used to describe all cases in which sclerotic changes occur in the arteries.

The development of atherosclerotic lesions does not lend itself easily to precise measurement in the living. However, the extent and severity of coronary atherosclerosis determines the risk of CHD in a given population.[4] *Coronary risk factors* are those abnormalities demonstrable in persons free of CHD and known to be associated with significantly increased risk of developing the disease in subsequent years.

Some information on risk factors was obtained from population surveys and from retrospective studies comparing patients with CHD against control groups similar in all other respects. The most convincing evidence of association of specific abnormalities with subsequent development of CHD has come from prospective surveys, for example, the Los Angeles Heart Study,[2] the Framingham Study,[5-8] the Albany Study,[9] and the Western Electric Company Study.[10] Such studies were designed to obtain an accurate measure of disease development in a defined population of initially clinically well people over a period of time. Accumulated results of these studies are most illuminating in that the susceptibility of an individual or a subgroup of the population to CHD can be assessed on an actuarial basis according to the risk factors present.

Prospective studies prove beyond all reasonable doubt that the risk of experiencing a clinical episode of CHD is a function of altered serum lipid and cholesterol levels.[11-13] Other risk factors include hypertension, diabetes mellitus, obesity, diet, cigarette smoking, physical inactivity, stress factors, positive family history, and a sex-related difference.

LIPIDS AND LIPOPROTEINS

The serum lipids are derived from both endogenous and exogenous sources and are absorbed, metabolized, transported, modified, and stored. It is now recognized that the major lipids in transport are component parts of complex lipoprotein molecules. Thus different amounts and types of protein and lipids combine to form the various types of lipoprotein.[14] Cholesterol, phospholipids, and triglycerides are the major lipid fractions in the blood.

Cholesterol   Cholesterol is the most abundant sterol, becoming a structural component of cells and plasma lipoproteins and the source of bile acids and steroid hormones. The circulating cholesterol is largely synthesized in the liver and discharged into plasma bound to lipoproteins. The plasma cholesterol pool reflects the net result of a series of reactions which are donating sterol to the pool while others are removing it.[15]

Numerous prospective studies on western populations have indicated a close correlation between the moiety with elevated cholesterol levels and their proneness to CHD.[1,5,7] Population groups with hypercholesterolemia experience four times as many heart attacks as those with low serum cholesterol levels.[16] This strong relationship is well shown in the Framingham Study,[5-7] and in the Los Angeles Heart Study.[2] Katz and Stamler[17] have demonstrated experimentally a similiar relationship. They noted that feeding cholesterol to cockerels produced coronary atherosclerosis.

Among western populations, serum cholesterol and other blood lipids rise with age.[18] Serum cholesterol is thought to increase from about 180 mg/100 ml between the ages of 20 and 30 years to about 220 between the ages of 50 and 60 years. The levels vary, however, in different population groups. For example, Barr[19] recorded mean levels of 197 in normal women aged 18 to 35, and 252 in normal women aged 45 to 65 years. Oliver and Boyd[20] reported mean levels of 217 for women aged 40 to 49 years, 240 for those aged 50 to 54 years, and 259 for those aged 55 to 59 years. The risks of coronary thrombosis are said to be seriously increased if serum cholesterol levels exceed 250.[5,13]

Cholesterol is a precursor of estrogenic hormones. Endogenous estrogens appear to influence cholesterol metabolism in at least two ways. There is an effect on the biosynthetic mechanism and also an influence on the rate of degradation or excretion.[15] Thus estrogens appear to exert an effect on human plasma cholesterol and lipidlipoprotein levels.

Phospholipids   Phospholipids, like cholesterol, are present in all cells and are abundant throughout the body. Most plasma phospholipids are derived from the liver. Their actual role in the plasma is not well understood. It was thought that they help stabilize less polar lipids like cholesterol and tryglicerides, that is, act as "biologic detergents." However, this ability is really the property of the apoproteins.[21]

Triglycerides   Triglycerides are esters of fatty acids and glycerol. They are absorbed from the intestine, stored in adipose tissue, and broken down by lipase into free fatty acids (FFA), also called nonesterified fatty acids (NEFA). The latter reaction is under hormonal influence; it is triggered by energy demands from the body.[14]

Lipoproteins   A major physical change occurs when lipids bind with proteins to form lipoproteins. The lipids which are water-insoluble attain the ability to remain dispersed in body fluids.[14,22,23]

There are four major classes of lipoproteins, which are usually classified as follows:

Ultracentrifugation	Electrophoresis
High density lipoproteins (HDL)	Alpha lipoproteins
Low density lipoproteins (LDL)	Beta lipoproteins
Very low density lipoproteins (VLDL) (endogenous)	Prebeta lipoproteins
Very low density lipoproteins (exogenous)	Chylomicrons

Lipid studies have generally emphasized that low-density lipoprotein and serum cholesterol have a positive correlation with CHD. In fact, serum cholesterol may be partitioned into high- and low-density lipoprotein fractions (HDL and LDL cholesterol, respectively). Recently an inverse relation has been found between CHD and serum HDL cholesterol.[24] The major lipid risk factor for CHD is probably a low concentration of serum HDL cholesterol.[25-27] For example, the increased incidence of coronary heart disease in women with diabetes mellitus has been associated with low serum HDL cholesterol concentrations.[28] On the other hand, children and adult populations free of CHD demonstrate high circulating HDL levels.[27] Norwegian skiers[29] and American runners[30] also have high HDL levels. Of practical relevance is the fact that concentrations of several circulating lipoproteins have been related to the severity of coronary atherosclerosis, HDL having an apparent retarding effect.[26]

An important question therefore needs to be addressed in decreasing the incidence of CHD and improving mortality statistics. This is to determine the specific relationship that exists between ovarian function, sex hormone, and lipoprotein concentrations, and the development of atherosclerosis and CHD.

RELATIONSHIP BETWEEN OVARIAN FUNCTION AND CHD

Some investigators have noted that the premenopausal female, compared with the human male, is protected against coronary accidents.[19,31,32] This sex difference is alleged to be due to estrogens. The evidence will be examined.

Evidence in Favor

Experimental and clinical data is available suggesting that endogenous ovarian estrogen secretion plays a key role in protecting women against clinical atherosclerotic coronary heart disease.

Numerous studies have been done on the effects of castration or premature menopause on the occurrence of both clinical heart disease and autopsy evidence of atherosclerosis in women.[19,33-36] Wuest et al. compared the degree of sclerosis in hearts of bilaterally oophorectomized women with hearts of men and women of comparable ages. They found that the degree of coronary sclerosis in the oophorectomized women was greater than in control women but less than in control men.[36]

Oliver and Boyd reported that bilateral oophorectomy was followed by the premature development of clinical coronary artery disease;[20] similar findings were found by Robinson et al.[35] Higano and Cohen reported the risk to be fourfold.[33] Novak and Williams[34] stated that the data of Robinson et al.[35] and Oliver and Boyd,[20] being clinical in nature, could not be as objective and precise as data obtained at autopsy. Regardless of initial age at operation or years intervening before death, they could find no significant differences in the incidence of atherosclerosis in statistically comparable groups of castrated and control patients at autopsy.[34] A follow-up study by the same investigators suggested that operation before the age of 40 might be of significance.[37]

Parrish et al. suspected that an important factor overlooked by previous writers was the time interval between castration and the expected age of the normal menopause. From a study of autopsy records they found that castrated patients did have an excess of coronary atherosclerosis and myocardial infarcts, but this was directly related to the time interval from castration to expected menopause and the time interval from castration to death. No excessive coronary atherosclerosis was found in women castrated after the age of 41, in contrast to those castrated when younger; excessive coronary atherosclerosis became apparent about 14 years after castration. They concluded that women castrated before the age of 40 who were expected to survive more than 14 years were at high risk of developing CHD.[38]

In a 6- to 20-year follow-up study of 35 women who had undergone spontaneous premature menopause, Sznajderman and Oliver further supported the view that cessation of ovarian activity, whether premature or at the time of a normal menopause, leads to an increase in the incidence of CHD and in serum-lipid levels in later life.[39]

Finally, the epidemiologic observations accumulating from the Framingham Study have done much to confirm the above clinical and pathological data. Women have about one-third the likelihood of men of developing a major cardiovascular event before reaching age 60. A biologic protective effect in women during their reproductive years is suggested by the fact that women have only about half the risk of men of the same age at any level of combined risk factors. Moreover, premenopausal women have only about one-third the risk of postmenopausal women of the same age (Table 6-1).[7,8]

Table 6-1. The Annual Incidence of Cardiovascular Disease (CHD, Brain Infarction, Congestive Failure) per Thousand Women According to Menopausal Status

Age	Premenopausal	Postmenopausal
40	0.6	2.2
40–44	0.6	3.6
45–49	2.0	4.0
50–54	3.6	6.5

Derived from the Framingham Study, Department of Health, Education and Welfare, Publication 74–599, 1974.

Evidence Against

Not all evidence has been positive in confirming a relationship between menopause status and the incidence of CHD. Utian reported a prospective investigation in statistically comparable groups of women, the only difference being the ovarian status. Oophorectomy was not shown to significantly increase the serum cholesterol value for at least two years after surgery.[40,41]

Despite the limitations of direct comparison, the summary in Table 6-2 is of interest. As can be seen in this table, the oophorectomized groups of Oliver and Boyd,[20] and of Utian,[40] and the normal women of the Barr[19] and Utian[40] studies demonstrate remarkably similar results. This lack of early direct response to endogenous estrogen withdrawal would therefore suggest estrogen to be of no more than secondary importance in the known relationship of increasing blood cholesterol with age.

Blanc et al. were unable to show a correlation between the age at menopause and the age of onset of myocardial infarction.[42] Moreover, selective coronary cinearteriography studies have failed to demonstrate any difference in amount of coronary atherosclerosis between surgically castrated women and control subjects.[43]

Rather than the ovaries having a protective effect against CHD, there have been several recent suggestions that it is the male sex hormones themselves that put the male in higher risk of developing CHD.[44,45] For instance, Phillips has reviewed evidence that males with myocardial infarction may have altered concentrations of estradiol to testosterone (E:T).[45,46] Specifically, he suggests that an increase in E:T may be the culprit in the pudgy, middle-aged man with mild diabetes, hyperlipidemia, and hypertension who appears prone to myocardial infarction.[45]

Support for this theory comes from Heller and Jacobs.[44] Their examination of mortality data in the United Kingdom suggested that women do not lose protection from CHD after menopause. Rather, around the age of 50, men begin to lose a factor that had previously put them at increased risk of developing CHD compared to women (Figure 6-1).

The tenuous nature of the association between an early menopause and CHD is confirmed by reevaluation of some of the original studies on which it was based.[47] The case control studies of castrated women comprised such different sorts of patients that variations in cardiovascular disease could easily be due to factors other than the presence or absence of ovaries.[20,35,38]

The Framingham Study can also not escape criticism.[6-8] Problems arise in interpreting the data. The report is based on a small number of events which include the historical development of angina, intermittent claudication, and congestive cardiac failure, as well as stroke and hard evidence of CHD (myocardial infarction and coronary death). When restricted to CHD deaths and myocardial infarction alone, there were only 31 events.[8] It is very difficult to draw conclusions on this small number.

Table 6-2. Comparative Findings in Several Studies of Serum Cholesterol Levels in Relation to Menopause Status

Author	Description	Age range (years)	Mean serum cholesterol ± S.D. (mg/100 ml)
Oliver and Boyd[20]	Bilateral oophorectomy 15–20 years previously	37–56	251 ± 43
Sznajderman and Oliver[39]	Spontaneous premature menopause 6–20 years previously	45–49	299
	Healthy women	45–49	217
Barr[19]	Normal women	45–65	252
Utian[40]	Normal premenopausal	45–55	268 ± 43
	Premenopausal immediately post-oophorectomy	45–55	250 ± 54
	2 years postoophorectomy	45–55	265 ± 41
	2 years posthysterectomy with conserved ovaries	45–55	260 ± 41

(From Utian: Int J Gynecol Obstet 10:95, 1972. Courtesy of Williams, Wilkins Co.)

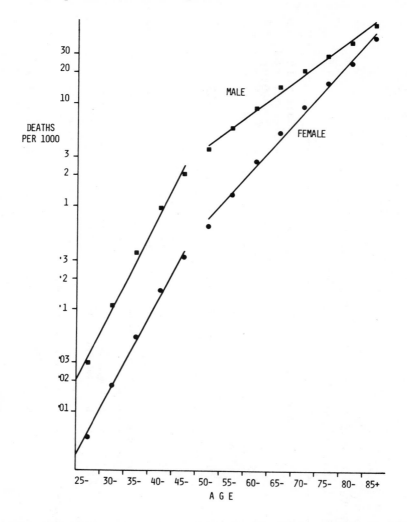

Figure 6–1.   Death rates from ischemic heart disease in men and women according to age (England and Wales, 1970–74). The change occurring at menopause is in men rather than in women. (From Heller and Jacobs: Br Med J 1:472, 1978. Courtesy of the British Medical Journal.)

EFFECTS OF EXOGENOUS ESTROGENS ON LIPIDS AND CHD

If the role of the functioning ovary in protecting against CHD appears tenuous, then the effects of estrogen therapy, on superficial evaluation at least, would suggest quite the reverse possibility. Once again, however, both sides of the coin need appraisal.

Early Positive Evidence

A wide range of estrogenic substances have been studied for their effects on cholesterol metabolism.[40,41,48,49,50] In the human, the administration of estrogenic substances at certain dosages was originally reported to depress the plasma cholesterol concentration,[20,50,51] although the dosage necessary to produce this effect was far in excess of the threshold estrogenic dose.[15,50]

Experimentally, estrogen administration was shown to inhibit coronary atherogenesis in cockerels fed a cholesterol-supplemented diet.[52] There are no comparable studies in man.

Oliver and Boyd administered estrogen to myocardial infarction survivors.[53] They found that although significant reduction of the serum-cholesterol was evident throughout the five years of treatment, the continued reduction of serum lipids did not improve prognosis once myocardial infarction had occurred. Similar findings were reported by Marmorston et al.[31] Numerous investigators have attempted to prove that exogenous estrogen therapy decreases the incidence of CHD, but there is no conclusive proof to date.[31,32,53,54,54A]

Despite the lack of definitive evidence, a growing tendency developed in the early 1960s toward the empirical use of long-term exogenous estrogen therapy in the postmenopausal woman as a preventive against CHD.[55-57] Particularly vociferous was the call from Wilson and Wilson for the maintenance of adequate estrogen from puberty to the grave.[58] Unfortunately, evidence was about to emanate from studies of estrogen in the oral contraceptive that these very drugs could possibly precipitate death.

Later Negative Evidence

Initial doubts about the safety of exogenous estrogens in relation to thromboembolic phenomena developed in 1968 when the oral contraceptive was identified as a risk factor for thromboembolic disease.[59] Moreover, the ability of estrogens to produce any significant depression of plasma cholesterol levels was questioned in a controlled prospective study.[40]

Then evidence appeared that taking hormones in the form of oral contraceptives increased the risk of developing CHD. The risk, as determined by three separate studies,[60-62] seems to be increased by between 2.8 and 4.7 times, depending on age. This risk was later suggested to occur almost exclusively in cigarette smokers on the oral contraceptive.[63]

Finally, early evidence from the Boston Collaborative Drug Surveillance Program has linked postmenopausal estrogen usage in young women with nonfatal myocardial infarction.[64] However, the case is weak, cigarette smokers again being the major subgroup at risk, and the same investigators in a larger study found no statistically significant association between current regular use of estrogens by older women and nonfatal acute myocardial infarction.[65]

Recent Estrogen and Lipid Studies

There are at least three possible reasons for the conflicting arguments presented above. These are the type of estrogen administered, the dosage selected, and the route of administration. Hopefully, an understanding of these factors may help unravel the as-yet unsolved enigma, i.e., how can the same hormones both protect from, and predispose toward, the same disease?

Type of Estrogen   The first possibility is that indeed these are not the same hormones.[40] Contraceptive pill studies almost without exception involve mixtures of ethinyl-estradiol (an alkyl substituted steroid) and various progestogens. For example, Arntzenius and co-workers in the Netherlands showed serum-HDL-cholesterol levels to be significantly higher in women aged 40 to 41 years then in men of the same age. Cigarette smoking and oral contraceptive use were both strongly associated with reduced serum-HDL-cholesterol. However, the contraceptive pill effect was independent of cigarette smoking and was a risk factor in itself. Pill users who smoked showed similar levels to men of the same age.[66] Several studies have confirmed this effect of the oral contraceptive and of ethinyl-estradiol in particular.[67]

On the other hand, Walter and Jensen could find no difference in blood lipids between patients treated with estradiol 2 mg, estriol 1 mg, or placebo.[68] These are so-called natural estrogens. Moreover, type II hypercholesterolemia has even been suggested as an indication for postmenopausal estrogens. Estradiol valerate, a conjugated estradiol ester, given to 17 women with this problem caused a depression of previously raised serum-LDL-cholesterol levels, and a 30 percent increase in previously depressed serum-HDL-cholesterol levels.[69] Estradiol valerate is rapidly metabolized to 17 β-estradiol, a natural human estrogen. Similar results have been reported in normal subjects treated with estradiol valerate[67] and conjugated equine estrogens.[70]

The evidence is thus suggestive that the natural estrogens induce different effects than the synthetic nonconjugated steroids. Considerable support for this theory comes from the many studies showing synthetic steroids to increase serum-triglyceride concentrations,[71] and the natural estrogens having virtually no such effect. Moreover, such studies indicate that the effects of estrogenic hormones on different lipoproteins are independent of each other.

Dosage   Not only is the type of estrogen of importance, but so may be the dose. Samsioe has confirmed the ability of 2 mg estradiol valerate to elevate HDL and reduce LDL, but at 4 mg dosage the pattern becomes the same as that for ethinyl-estradiol.[67] This area is in need of further research.

Route of Administration   Finally, a third factor may determine the lipid and lipoprotein response to estrogen. This is the route of administration of the drug. Percutaneous administration of estrogen apparently does not induce any change in blood triglyceride levels.[72] The reason for this difference can be explained by the elimination of the first liver passage of estrogens associated with oral absorption. Here, too, is an area in need of further study.

CONCLUSION

The long-term consequences of estrogens on lipid and lipoprotein metabolism are complex and incompletely understood at the present time. Initial optimism for a protective effect of the functioning ovary against the development of CHD is no longer so strong. A counter-argument is developing for the presence of a risk factor in the male that becomes less with age, rather than the female having a protective factor. In fact, both theories may have some validity and one should not exclude the other.

The possibility that the functioning ovary exerts some protective effect, however small, is a sound argument against the pernicious operation of bilateral oophorectomy in young females. A plea is therefore made for conservatism with normal ovaries during gynecologic surgery in young women.

Enough evidence does exist for questioning the empirical use of estrogens for the prevention of CHD in all women after the menopause. This does not mean that estrogens need be unduly withheld without valid reason. However, when estrogens are selected for postmenopausal use, due consideration should be given to type, dose, and route of administration.

The most urgent research need is to clarify the effects in postmenopausal women of all currently available estrogens, singly and in combination with other estrogens and progestogens. The development of new steroids with more specific effects is also possible, but entrance into the clinical area is not likely in the near future.

Somewhere in this enigma of varying hormone profiles with pre- and postmenopausal, and male and female differences may yet lie the key to understanding the etiology and prevention of CHD.

References

1.   Katz LN, Stamler J, Pick R: Nutrition and Atherosclerosis. Philadelphia, Lea and Febiger, 1958

2.   Chapman JM, Massey FJ: The inter-relationship of serum cholesterol, hypertension, body weight and coronary heart disease. The Los Angeles heart study. J Chronic Dis 17:933, 1964

3.   Bleyl U, Wegener K: Some current views on arteriosclerosis and its origins. Triangle 9:9, 1969

4.   McGill HC, Geer JC, Strong JP: Natural History of Human Atherosclerotic Lesions. New York, Academic, 1963

5.   Kannel WB, Dawber TR, Kagan A, Revotskie N, Stokes J: Factors of risk in the development of coronary heart disease — six year follow-up experience — the Framingham study. Ann Intern Med 55:33, 1961

6.   Kannel WB, Hjortland MC, McNamara PM, Gordon T: Menopause and risk of cardiovascular disease. The Framingham study. Ann Intern Med 85:447, 1976

7.   Shurtleff D: Some characteristics related to the incidence of cardiovascular disease and death: Framingham study, 18 year follow up. In Kannel WB, Gordon T (eds): The Framingham Study, Section 30. Washington, DC, Department of Health, Education and Welfare publication 74-599, 1974

8.   Gordon T, Kannel WB, Hjortland MC, McNamara PM: Menopause and coronary heart disease. The Framingham study. Ann Intern Med 89:157, 1978

9.   Doyle JT: Risk factors in coronary heart disease. NY State J Med 63:1317, 1963

10.   Paul O, Lepper MH, Phelan WH, et al.: A longitudinal study of coronary artery disease. Circulation 28:20, 1963

11.   Glueck CJ, Fallat RW: The heritable lipoproteinemias and atherosclerosis. Adv Exp Med Biol 63:305, 1975

12.   Oliver MF: Cholesterol, coronaries, clofibrate and death. N Engl J Med 299:1360, 1978

13.   Committee of Principal Investigators: A cooperative trial in the prevention of ischaemic heart disease using clofibrate. Br Heart J 40:1069, 1978

14.   Tall AR, Small DM: Plasma high-density lipoproteins. N Engl J Med 299:1232, 1978

15.   Boyd GS: Hormones and cholesterol metabolism. Biochem Soc Symp 24:79, 1963

16.   Stamler J: Atherosclerotic coronary heart disease — the major challenge to contemporary public health and preventive medicine. Conn Med 28:675, 1966

17.   Katz LN, Stamler J: Experimental Atherosclerosis. Springfield, Illinois, Thomas, 1953, p 291

18.   National Center for Health Statistics: Serum cholesterol level of adults, United States 1960-1962. Series II, No. 23. Washington, DC, Department Health, Education, Welfare, 1966

19.   Barr DP: Some chemical factors in the pathogenesis of atherosclerosis. Circulation 8:641, 1953

20.   Oliver MF, Boyd GS: Effect of bilateral ovariectomy on coronary-artery disease and serum-lipid levels. Lancet 2:690, 1959

21.   Tall AR, Small DM, Deckelbaum JH, et al.: Structure and thermodynamic properties of high density lipoprotein recombinants. J Biol Chem 252:4701, 1977

22.   Berger GMB: HDL in the prevention of arteriosclerotic heart disease. Part I, epidemiological and family studies. S Afr Med J 54:689, 1978

23.   Berger GMB: HDL in the prevention of atherosclerotic heart disease. Part II, biochemical role in the pathogenesis of atherosclerosis. S Afr Med J 54:693, 1978

24.   Castelli WP, Doyle JT, Gordon T, et al.: HDL cholesterol and other lipids in coronary heart disease. The cooperative lipoprotein phenotyping study. Circulation 55:767, 1977

25.   Miller GJ, Miller NW: Plasma high-density-lipoprotein concentration and development of ischemic heart disease. Lancet 1:16, 1975

26.   Jenkins PJ, Harper RW, Nestel PJ: Severity of coronary atherosclerosis related to lipoprotein concentration. Br Med J 2:388, 1978

27.   Walker ARP, Walker BF: High high-density-lipoprotein cholesterol in African children and adults in a population free of coronary heart disease. Br Med J 2:1336, 1978

28.   Gordon T, Castelli WP, Hjortland MC, Kannel WB, Dawber TR: Diabetes, blood lipids, and the role of obesity in coronary heart disease risk for women. Ann Intern Med 87:393, 1977

29.   Enger SC, Herbjornsen K, Erikssen J, Fretland A: High density lipoprotein (HDL) and physical activity: the influence of physical exercise, age and smoking on HDL-cholesterol and the HDL/total cholesterol ratio. Scand J Clin Lab Invest 37:251, 1977

30.   Hulley SB, Cohen R, Widdowson G: Plasma high-density lipoprotein cholesterol level. Influence of risk factor intervention. JAMA 238:2269, 1977

31.   Marmorston J, Moore FJ, Hopkins CE, Kuzma OT, Weiner J: Clinical studies of long-term estrogen therapy in men with myocardial infarction. Proc Soc Exp Biol Med 110:400, 1962

32.   Stamler J, Pick R, Katz LN, et al.: Effectiveness of estrogens for the therapy of myocardial infarction in middle-aged men. JAMA 183:632, 1963

33.   Higano RW, Cohen WD: Increased incidence of cardiovascular disease in castrated women. Med Intelligence 268:1123, 1963

34.   Novak ER, Williams TJ: Autopsy comparison of cardiovascular changes in castrated and normal women. Am J Obstet Gynecol 80:863, 1960

35.   Robinson RW, Higano N, Cohen WS: Increased incidence of coronary heart disease in women castrated prior to the menopause. Arch Intern Med 104:908, 1959

36.   Wuest JH, Dry TJ, Edwards JE: The degree of coronary atherosclerosis in bilaterally oophorectomized women. Circulation 7:801, 1953

37.   Williams TJ, Novak ER: Effects of castration and hysterectomy on the female cardiovascular system. Geriatrics 18:852, 1963

38.   Parrish HM, Carr CA, Hall DG, King TM: Time interval from castration in premenopausal women to development of excessive coronary atherosclerosis. Am J Obstet Gynecol 99:155, 1967

39.   Sznajderman M, Oliver MF: Spontaneous premature menopause, ischaemic heart disease, and serum lipids. Lancet 1:962, 1963

40.   Utian WH: Effects of oophorectomy and estrogen therapy on serum cholesterol. Int J Gynecol Obstet 10:95, 1972

41.   Utian WH: Cholesterol, coronary heart disease and oestrogens. S Afr Med J 45:359, 1971

42.   Blanc J, Boschat J, Morin J, Clavier J, Penther P: Menopause and myocardial infarction. Am J Obstet Gynecol 127:353, 1977

43.   Manchester JH, Herman MV, Gorlin R: Premenopausal castration and documented coronary atherosclerosis. Am J Cardiol 28:34, 1971

44.   Heller RJ, Jacobs HS: Coronary heart disease in relation to age, sex, and the menopause. Br Med J 1:472, 1978

45.   Phillips GB: Sex hormones, risk factors and cardiovascular disease. Am J Med 65:7, 1978

46.   Phillips GB: Relationship between serum sex hormones and glucose, insulin, and lipid abnormalities in men with myocardial infarction. Proc Natl Acad Sci USA 74:1729, 1977

47.   Editorial: Coronary heart disease and the menopause. Br Med J 1:862, 1977

48.   Drill VA, Riegel B: Structural and hormonal activity of some new steroids. Recent Prog Horm Res 14:29, 1958

49.   Nestel PJ, Hirsch EZ, Couzens EA: The effect of chlorophenoxyisobutyric acid and ethinyl estradiol on cholesterol turnover. J Clin Invest 44:891, 1965

50.   Robinson RW, Higano N, Cohen WD: Effects of long-term administration of estrogens on serum lipids of postmenopausal women. N Engl J Med 263:828, 1960

51.   Davis ME, Jones RJ, Jarolim C: Long-term estrogen substitution and atherosclerosis. Am J Obstet Gynecol 82:1003, 1961

52.   Pick R, Stamler J, Rodbard S, Katz LN: The inhibition of coronary atherosclerosis by estrogens in cholesterol-fed chicks. Circulation 6:276, 1952

53.   Oliver MF, Boyd GS: Influence of reduction of serum-lipids on prognosis of coronary heart disease. A five-year study using oestrogen. Lancet 2:499, 1961

54.   Spritz N: Atherosclerosis and the menopause. Mod Treat 5:581, 1968

54A.   Hammond CB, Jelovsek FR, Lee KL, et al.: Effect of long-term estrogen replacement therapy. I. Metabolic effects. Am J Obstet Gynecol 133:525, 1979

55.   Davis ME, Jones RJ, Jarolim C: Long-term estrogen substitution and atherosclerosis. Am J Obstet Gynecol 82:1003, 1961

56.   Davis ME: Long-term estrogen substitution after the menopause. Clin Obstet Gynecol 7:558, 1964

57.   McEwen DC: Ovarian failure and the menopause. J Can Med Assoc 92:962, 1965

58.   Wilson RA, Wilson TA: The fate of non-treated postmenopausal women. A plea for the maintenance of adequate estrogen from puberty to the grave. J Am Geriatr Soc 11:347, 1963

59.   Inman WHW, Vessey MP: Investigation of deaths from pulmonary, coronary and cerebral thrombosis and embolism in women of child-bearing age. Br Med J 2:193, 1968

60.   Mann JI, Vessey MP, Thorogood M, et al.: Myocardial infarction in young women with special reference to oral contraceptive practice. Br med J 2:241, 1975

61.   Mann JI, Inman WHW: Oral contraceptives and death from myocardial infarction. Br Med J 2:245, 1975

62.   Royal College of General Practitioners: Mortality among oral-contraceptive users, Royal College of General Practitioners Oral Contraception Study. Lancet 2:727, 1977

63.   Jick H, Dinan B, Rothman KJ: Noncontraceptive estrogens and nonfatal myocardial infarction. JAMA 239:1407, 1978

64.   Jick H, Dinan B, Rothman KJ: Noncontraceptive estrogens and nonfatal myocardial infarction. JAMA 239:1407, 1978

65.   Rosenberg L, Armstrong B, Jick H: Myocardial infarction and estrogen therapy in post-menopausal women. N Engl J Med 294:1256, 1976

66.   Arntzenius AC, van Gent CM, van der Voort H, et al.: Reduced high-density lipoprotein in women aged 40-41 using oral contraceptives. Lancet 1:1221, 1978

67.   Samsioe G: Workshop on metabolic effects of the menopause. Utian WH (moderator). In van Keep PA (ed): Female and Male Climacteric. Lancaster, MTP Press, 1979, p 95

68.   Walker S, Jensen HK: The effect of treatment with oestradiol and oestriol on fasting serum cholesterol and triglyceride levels in postmenopausal women. Br J Obstet Gynaecol 84:869, 1977

69.   Tikkanen MJ, Nikkila EA, Vartiainen E: Natural oestrogen as an effective treatment for type-II hyperlipoproteinaemia in postmenopausal women. Lancet 2:491, 1978

70.   Roth MS, Donato DM, Lansman HH, et al.: Effects of steroids on serum lipids and serum cholesterol binding reserve. Am J Obstet Gynecol 132:151, 1978

71.   Wallentin L, Varenhorst E: Changes of plasma lipid metabolism in males during estrogen treatment for prostatic carcinoma. J Clin Endocrinol Metab 47:596, 1978

72.   Loeper J, Loeper J, Ohlgiessr C, de Lignieres B, Mauvais-Jarvis P: The influence of estrogen therapy on triglycerides. Importance of the choice of substance and the route of administration. Nouv Presse Med 6:2747, 1977

7
Symptom Formation

Early in the summer of 1976, the First International Congress on Menopause was convened at La Grande Motte, near Montpellier, in southern France. One of the first objectives facing the meeting, held under the auspices of the International Health Foundation, the American Geriatric Society, and the University of Montpellier, was to classify the symptomatology associated with climacteric.

The difficult task of definition was accomplished with the cooperation of a panel of international authorities under the chairmanship of Utian and Serr.[1] The consensus reached at that meeting was as follows:

1. The climacteric is that phase in the aging process of women marking the transition from the reproductive stage of life to the nonreproductive stage.
2. Menopause indicates the final menstrual period and occurs during the climacteric. Present estimations date this at about 51 years.
3. The climacteric is sometimes, but not necessarily always, associated with symptomatology. When this occurs it may be termed the "climacteric syndrome."

Climacteric symptoms and complaints are derived from three main components:

1. Decreased ovarian activity with subsequent hormonal deficiency resulting in early symptoms (hot flushes, perspiration, and atrophic vaginitis), and late symptoms related to the metabolic change in the end organ affected.
2. Sociocultural factors determined by the woman's environment.
3. Psychologic factors, dependent on the structure of the woman's character.

The variety of symptomatology is the result of interaction between these three components.*

*From Utian and Serr: The climacteric syndrome. In Van Keep, Greenblatt, and Albeaux-Fernet (eds): Consensus on Menopause Research. Lancaster, 1976, p. 1. Courtest of MTP Press.

BACKGROUND TO SYMPTOM PRODUCTION

Until the early 1970s it was extremely difficult to come to any conclusion regarding the true symptoms associated with climacteric. Symptoms of any type were usually divided on an empirical basis into "autonomic," "psychologic," and "metabolic," or else simply itemized grocery-list style without any attempt at explanation. Investigators often had difficulty understanding each others' lines of research. Clinicians were really in the dark as to causation of symptoms, and were inevitably forced to treat effect on an empirical basis rather than cause on a valid scientific basis.

The problem was a lack of established scientific data relating to human climacteric. Even much of the published research showed serious deficiencies in patient sampling and methodology.[2] In particular, there was virtually no published information relating specific symptoms or signs with parameters of estrogen production or secretion. Other notable deficiencies included the real clinical changes related specifically to postmenopausal endocrine profiles, the early and late effects of bilateral oophorectomy, and the clinical use of exogenous estrogens, particularly in separating true drug effects from placebo responses. Finally, there was minimal information on the psychologic and sociocultural contributions to symptom formation. The majority of clinical features ascribed to this period in the human life cycle were therefore mere assumptions, and could have been no more than coincidental features in a generally aging population.

A virtual flurry of publications from 1970 onward did much to remedy the lack of specific data.[3-15] This is not to decry the attempts of earlier investigators in defining menopausal symptomatology, but rather to state that invariably case selection, controls, or empirical scoring systems were not specific enough to provide the required information.[16-19]

While further clarification is necessary,[15] the International Classification does help clear up confusion. The definitive statement is made that the varied symptom profile after menopause is caused by an interaction between three components: (1) decreased ovarian activity with altered hormone profiles, (2) sociocultural or environmental factors, and (3) psychologic factors.

Prior to considering these three components further, one aspect should be emphasized. The classification allows for the fact that the nature and incidence of symptomatology varies in different educational, socioeconomic, racial, and population groups. But it lays stress on the actual causal agent of the symptom, thus suggesting that treatment must be selective. For instance, hormone-dependent symptoms will be best treated by appropriate hormonal replacement; other symptoms may justify psychotherapy or actual educational programs to alter negative attitudes in specific sociocultural groups. The logic of this will become clearer once the above three causative mechanisms have been reviewed.

There is in the literature little information concerning the number of women who have sufficient symptoms at the time of the menopause to seek medical advice. A statistical study of 1000 women in England indicated that 15.8 percent had no symptoms at the time of the menopause, 62.3 percent had only hot flushes for an average duration of two years, and 89.7 percent carried on their daily activities without interruption.[20] Although it is reported that as many as 75 percent of women have distressful symptoms at the menopause,[21] it is more generally agreed that 10 to 15 percent of women will present themselves for medical advice for symptoms attributed to the climacteric.[10,13,18,22,23] It is apparent from the foregoing discussion, however, that these figures mean rather little, and will vary according to the population actually surveyed.

SPECIFIC HORMONE-RELATED SYMPTOMS

The information presented in Chapters Three through Six makes this section fairly self-explanatory. That is, target organ responses to altered hormone profiles after menopause are relatively specific. In certain instances, these tissue changes are pathologic and will be severe enough to evoke a symptom, and in a variable percentage of these the symptom will be severe enough to become a complaint that is taken to the physician.

The actual symptoms that are specifically related to hormonal changes are conveniently subdivided according to the time of onset. This concept of one syndrome occurring over a period of time has been well described by van Keep and Kellerhals and is schematically summarized in Figure 7-1.[24]

Early Symptoms

AMMENORRHEA AND MENSTRUAL IRREGULARITY   The one definite feature of the climacteric is the menopause, that is, permanent secondary amenorrhea. Prior to this event there can be an alteration in the menstrual cycle with irregularity of periods, increase in length of cycle, or a decrease in flow.[18] Prolonged intervals between menstrual bleeding are probably due to the relative scarcity of follicles suitable for the gonadotropin-dependent final stages of follicular development.[25]

Some women have unusually short cycles before menopause.[26] These may result from either a decrease in the length of the follicular phase[25] or from defective luteal function.[27]

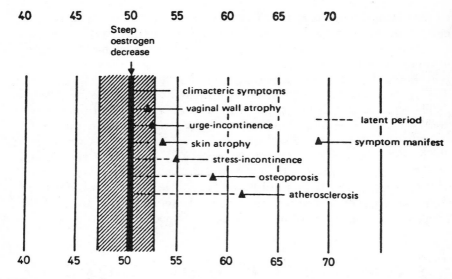

Figure 7-1.   Symptoms of estrogen deficiency and age; a schematic representation of the climacteric as one syndrome occurring over a period of time. (From van Keep and Kellerhals: Front Horm Res 2:160, 1973. Courtesy of Karger Publishers.)

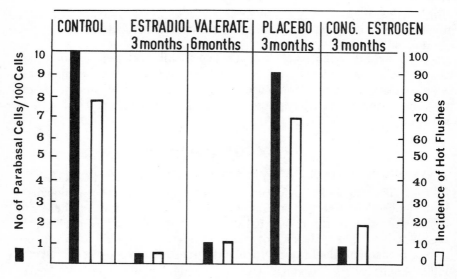

Figure 7-2.   The significant relationship between the vaginal parabasal cell index and the incidence of hot flushes in 50 oophorectomized patients on estrogen and placebo therapy. (From Utian: Front Horm Res 3:74, 1975. Courtesy of Karger Publishers.)

Alterations in the amount of bleeding will depend upon the endometrial response to the above factors.

HOT FLUSHES (FLASHES)   It is most likely that the only other actual early symptom resulting from diminished ovarian activity, apart from amenorrhea, is the vasomotor instability that manifests as hot flushes.[3,4,6]

The flush is usually described as a sudden feeling of heat in the face, neck, and chest, associated with diffuse or patchy flushing of the skin or perspiration. Vasodilatation is followed by vasoconstriction, so after a flush comes a cold shiver. The flush is a manifestation of vasomotor instability and is brought on particularly by excitement or nervousness. It can occur at any time of the day or night, the latter often termed "night sweats."

The hot flush is the one symptom allowing definite measurement in that the patient is usually able to describe the number of hot flushes suffered per twenty-four-hour period. Thus the incidence of the symptom can be compared under different circumstances.

Utian reported a comparative controlled prospective study in which a wide spectrum of symptoms was analyzed in normal pre- and postmenopausal patients, and in patients undergoing hysterectomy with and without removal of ovaries.[3,4,6] There was a low incidence of hot flushes in patients undergoing hysterectomy with conservation of ovaries, and this incidence did not significantly increase for at least two years after such surgery, i.e., the conserved ovaries continued to function for at least two years. Following oophorectomy there was a highly significant increase in the incidence of this symptom, 50 percent of patients having flushes. Comparison of the oophorectomized with the nonoophorectomized group revealed highly significant differences (p < 0.001). Retention of ovaries decreased the likelihood of the development of hot flushes.[6]

Utian also correlated the parabasal cell index with the severity of numerous symptoms.[6,28] Hot flushes were the only symptom to show a positive correlation (Figure 7-2).

The response of hot flushes to estradiol valerate and conjugated estrogen administration was striking (p < 0.001), with relief of the symptoms in the majority of patients. This cure is not a placebo effect, as single-blind crossover to placebo resulted in return of the symptoms in a high proportion of cases (66 percent), and this finding was highly significant (p < 0.001). Both forms of estrogen used in this study were effective (p < 0.001) and no statistical difference in effect between the two hormones could be demonstrated. Thus, the symptom of hot flushes was shown to be estrogen-dependent. Perspiration (night sweats) followed

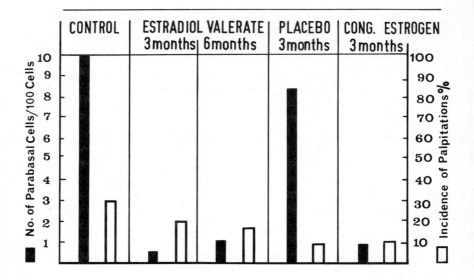

Figure 7–3.   Relationship between parabasal cell index and the incidence of palpitations in 50 oophorectomized patients. The placebo response of palpitations to estrogen and placebo therapy is well demonstrated. (From Utian: Front Horm Res 3:74, 1975. Courtesy of Karger Publishers.)

much the same pattern as hot flushes. However, a placebo effect is well illustrated for palpitations in Figure 7-3.

The conclusion that the hot flush and associated perspiration is the only early symptom directly resulting from hormone withdrawal following oophorectomy and, by analogy, the normal climacteric, is well substantiated in the medical literature.[13,18,29,30]

The mechanism of flushing has not been elucidated. The long popular theory that flushes are due to increased gonadotropins is no longer acceptable.[31] Nor does flushing appear to be related to particular concentrations of plasma estrone, estradiol, or androstenedione levels.[15] This does not exclude the likelihood of a declining level of estrogen being responsible for the flushing response; that is, a changing state rather than an absolute state. But this theory, too, remains to be tested. It may explain why flushes can occur before the menopause.

Sturdee and co-workers have reported the onset of the hot flush to be associated with a sudden and transient increase in sympathetic drive.[32] This finding has been disputed.[33] Hutton et al. have suggested that the catechol-estrogens may be involved, but this too is unproven.[15] Flushing is associated with endogenous adrenergic discharge and exogenous catecholamines.[34] Further research along this line will hopefully solve this puzzle in the near future and perhaps result in suitable alternatives to estrogen for treatment.

flushing = Kid Yin Xu → Kid Fire.

Later Symptoms

The production of later postmenopausal symptoms is more complex. Target organ responses to changing endocrine profiles were discussed in depth previously (Chapter 4). Inevitably, symptoms and signs can result from the metabolic derangements that occur in the specific target tissues. Thus atrophic (senile) vaginitis, for example, may produce symptoms of dyspareunia or pruritus vulvae. Some other possible symptoms developing on the basis of this mechanism can be summarized as follows:

Target Organ	Possible Symptom
Vulva and vagina	Dyspareunia ? Bloodstained discharge Pruritus vulvae
Bladder and urethra	Frequency and/or urgency Stress incontinence
Uterus and pelvic floor	Utero-vaginal prolapse
Skin and mucous membranes	Dryness or pruritus Easily traumatized Loss of resilience and pliability Dry hair or loss of hair Minor hirsutism of face Dry mouth Voice changes — reduction in upper register
Cardiovascular system	Angina and CHD
Skeleton	Fracture of hip and wrist Backache
Breasts	Reduced size Softer consistency Drooping

If the climacteric syndrome is recognized as a continuous one developing over several years, then it can be accepted that the clinical presentation could involve one or several of the above symptoms. Recognition of the problem could be complicated by specific patient idiosyncracies. For instance, the elderly woman with painful intercourse may be hesitant to voice such a problem directly and complain instead of something else. There are, moreover, other symptoms not caused by altered hormone profiles that may be just as real to the patient and with which she could present.

PSYCHOLOGIC COMPONENT
OF SYMPTOM PRODUCTION

The host of other symptoms such as palpitations, fatigue, vertigo, headaches, dyspnea, irritability, depression, frigidity, and apprehension that are listed as components of the climacteric syndrome are probably manifestations of the psychologic disturbances that may occur at this time of life and there is no evidence that these symptoms are causally related to altered hormone profiles.[24,35] There is also no evidence that libido is affected by menopause, although it is possible that hysterectomy may deleteriously affect this function.[36]

The actual verification and classification of these symptoms within the sphere of climacteric has proven exceptionally difficult. Not only do social and ethnic differences exist,[37] but outside influences such as work and play also modify responses to climacteric.[38] Above all, it has been almost impossible to define the problem and to undertake inter-study or cross-cultural comparisons because of the lack of adequate tools to measure changes in behavior. For example, the gynecologist refers to postmenopausal depression but really understands this as an altered mood up to the point where normal behavior ends and clinical depression begins. The psychiatrist, on the other hand, has a different perception of the problem.

Fortunately, adequate tools are becoming available for measuring marginal changes in behavior and responses to stressful situations or different forms of treatment.[39-42] Application of such specific measures has helped clarify areas in need of further investigation. Similarly, it has been possible to demonstrate that certain psychologic symptoms do occur with increased frequency in relationship to climacteric. The psychologic component of menopause has been recently reviewed by Dennerstein and Burrows[43] and by Brown and Brown.[44]

Types of Psychiatric Symptoms

It is generally accepted that climacteric does not precipitate any major psychiatric illness.[44] The following psychologic symptoms have been reported with climacteric:[43,44]

Fatigue or diminished drive
Vertigo (dizziness)
Irritability
Apprehension
Insomnia
Altered libido
Feeling of inadequacy or
    nonfulfillment

Loss of ability to concentrate
    or apathy
Headache
Depression
Tension or anxiety
Dyspnea
General fluctuations in mood

Unfortunately a list such as this contains many vague and ill-defined terms, most of which are not exclusive to psychiatric problems, but could occur in organic illnesses where no psychiatric disorder is suspected.[44]

Causes of Psychiatric Symptoms

Minor psychiatric symptoms occur on a multifactorial basis, the elucidation of which needs individualized diagnosis. The following are but a few of the factors that can be involved.[11,43-46]

Age of onset of menopause, marital status, parity, occupation, and educational and income status are factors of immediate importance. The ability shown at a younger age to adjust to difficulties in general will influence responses to the events of aging. Attitudes toward menstruation and toward the female role are also of significance.

Van Keep and Prill have suggested that distinguishing reaction patterns exist and can be demonstrated in a population of menopausal age.[11] They describe four different ways of reacting to menopause:

1. The passive reaction is a passive acceptance of the inevitable, usually found in women with limited intelligence or from rural communities.
2. The neurotic reaction is an extreme reaction triggered by resistance to the aging process and manifesting as nervousness, depression, or irritability.
3. The hyperactive reaction is a refusal to recognize the situation, manifesting with an intense interest in careers or hobbies, and marked criticism of women who complain.
4. The adequate reaction is a satisfactory adjustment which is shown by the majority of women.[11]

EPIDEMIOLOGIC STUDIES   The methodologic problems in surveying the incidence and cause of psychiatric symptoms were mentioned previously. The most important are unsatisfactory descriptions of the type of patient studied and her menopause status, biased sampling in that often select groups are sampled and not random populations, retrospective instead of prospective studies, inadequate definition and measure of symptoms, etc. It is not surprising, therefore, that any survey of the current psychiatric literature uncovers a number of inconsistencies.[43] Nonetheless, a general trend confirming an increased perimenopausal frequency of the above-listed minor psychiatric symptoms does exist,[10,24,43,47-50] although not all authors are in agreement.[45,46,51,52] The response to these symptoms can be profoundly influenced by social and cultural differences.

SOCIOCULTURAL INFLUENCE ON SYMPTOM FORMATION

It is incorrect to view climacteric on a purely biologic basis. The response to menopause is modified by many factors, one important one being the sociocultural environment.[37,53]

Thus, the individual will develop symptoms in response to the target-tissue changes and the psychologic components described above. But the society in which a women lives and moves, works and plays, is of paramount importance to the way in which she will adjust to menopause. The environment in which the female finds herself during the time of menopause will have a considerable influence on the way she responds to any symptoms she may develop. In many instances, a mild symptom may become a moderate one, or a symptom she can live with becomes a complaint that she takes to her physician.

In simple terms, some societies reward women for having reached menopause or the end of the fertile period, while others in effect actually punish them.[52] Many examples come to mind. In some African tribes the women after menopause graduate from being "bearers of children and drawers of water" to full tribal equality. They can sit in on the tribal council and participate in decision making, and in effect become full-fledged members of the "tribal parliament." Another striking illustration of this cultural attitude is shown with women of the Rahjput classes in India.[53] They experience few symptoms and look forward to menopause because they emerge from Purdah at the end of their childbearing years. That is, they no longer are required to wear a veil and acquire higher status because they are not "contaminated" by menstrual blood. A similar situation has been described for certain Arab women for whom the end of the fertile period brings positive changes in their lives.[37]

On the other hand, in most Western societies there is a strong emphasis on a youth-oriented culture. Being "young and beautiful" becomes a matter of prime concern; cosmetics, mode of dress, and the correct youthful image become important. Women from such societies see nothing positive about menopause, only a reminder that they are no longer young.[54]

Other stresses are added to the above problem around the age of menopause. The average woman at age 50 may find a change of social status, lose one or both parents, lose her children to college or marriage, and she may become a mother-in-law, a grandmother, or both. Her husband may stray or become ill. These are all social components that are liable to produce psychologic stresses dependent on the basic character of the women affected.[11,54]

Studies have shown that important alternate roles at the time of menopause, for example, a profession, or being the sole wage earner, lessen the symptom profile of climacteric.[11] However, the matter is more complicated and additional factors such as general health and stability and marital relationships are involved.[37] For this reason Maoz et al. feel the advice "to go out and work" which is so often given to menopausal women is not always correct, and should not be given automatically.[38] Each woman should be evaluated individually for her specific psychobiologic and sociocultural background.

The menopausal woman's interpretation of herself, her role model, is thus of importance. Large-scale educational programs are necessary to explain positive attitudes and improve what is often an incorrect image. Before this can be successfully achieved, a number of areas still need elucidation. These include such aspects as the influence of menopause on marital relations and vice versa, the specific problems of the single woman (unmarried, divorced or widowed), the effects of sex education, longitudinal studies with and without therapy, and so on.[53] Certainly, far more attention needs to be directed at the sociocultural aspects of menopause and much more recognition given to its role in the overall mechanism of symptom production.

SEXUAL FUNCTION AFTER MENOPAUSE

Knowledge about sexual function and sexual response after menopause is less than satisfactory. The perpetuation of a number of myths about sex in aging populations has resulted in unsatisfactory stereotyping and negative attitudes. In a remarkably forthright review, Kuhn has listed some of these myths, including "sex doesn't matter in old age," "interest in sex is abnormal for old people" and "remarriage after loss of spouse should be discouraged."[55] The belief that sexual response is reduced in the postmenopausal woman is a cultural fallacy. Climacteric in itself appears to have little effect on sex function.[4,56] Painful intercourse as a complication of vaginal atrophy is a cause of dyspareunia, not true loss of libido. In fact, it has been shown that removal of normally functioning ovaries from premenopausal women does not affect libido unless the uterus itself is removed.[7] Even the latter is most probably associated with psychologic factors due to inadequate preoperative patient counseling.[56] It is therefore not unexpected that estrogen replacement therapy after menopause has been shown to be of no benefit in the treatment of decreased or absent libido[7] unless specifically associated with dyspareunia.[3,4,6,56]

CONCLUSION

Critical review of the medical literature leads to the conclusion that the climacteric, whether artificial or spontaneous, is associated with certain specific symptoms.[35] Contrary to popular opinion, however, the number and variety of direct, true hormonal-related effects are less than generally assumed. The following classification of perimenopausal symptoms summarizes current thought and, being practical, is easily related to the clinical situation:

1. Specific: True hormonal-related symptoms
   Early: hot flushes; perspiration (night sweats)
   Later: relate to the metabolic change in the target organ affected; e.g., osteoporosis causing backache, vaginal atrophy causing dyspareunia, etc.
2. Nonspecific: Psycho-socio-cultural symptoms
   Determined by the woman's environment and the structure of her character; e.g., depression, irritability, insomnia, frigidity, headache, apprehension, etc.

It therefore follows that a case can be made for hormonal treatment of specific symptoms but not for the nonspecific ones. The details of therapy are subjects for discussion in the chapters that follow.

References

1. Utian WH, Serr D: The climacteric syndrome. In van Keep, Greenblatt, Albeaux-Fernet (eds): Consensus on Menopause Research. Lancaster, MTP Press, 1976, p. 1

2. McKinlay SM, McKinlay JB: Selected studies of the menopause. J Biosoc Sci 5:533, 1973

3. Utian WH: Clinical and metabolic effects of the menopause and the role of replacement oestrogen therapy. Unpublished Ph. D. Thesis, University of Cape Town, 1970

4. Utian WH: The true clinical features of postmenopause and oophorectomy, and their response to oestrogen therapy. S Afr Med J 46:732, 1972

5. Utian WH: The mental tonic effect of oestrogens administered to oophorectomized females. S Afr Med J 46:1079, 1972

6. Utian WH: Definitive symptoms of postmenopause — incorporating use of vaginal parabasal cell index. Front Horm Res 3:74, 1975

7. Utian WH: Effect of hysterectomy, oophorectomy and estrogen therapy on libido. Int J Gynaecol Obstet 13:97, 1975

8.   Utian WH: The scientific basis for postmenopausal estrogen therapy. The management of specific symptoms and rationale for long-term replacement. In Beard R (ed): The Menopause. Lancaster, MTP Press, 1976, p. 175

9.   Stone SC, Mickal A, Rye PH: Postmenopausal symptomatology, maturation index and plasma estrogen levels. Obstet Gynecol 45:625, 1975

10.   Jaszmann L: Epidemiology of climacteric and postclimacteric complaints. Front Horm Res 2:22, 1973

11.   van Keep PA, Prill HJ: Psycho-sociology of menopause and post-menopause. Front Horm Res 3:32, 1975

12.   Kruskemper G: Results of psychological testing (MMPI) in climacteric women. Front Horm Res 3:105, 1975

13.   Thompson B, Hart HA, Durno S: Menopausal age and symptomatology in a general practice. J Biosoc Sci 5:71, 1973

14.   Abe T, Furuhashi N, Yamaya Y, et al.: Correlation between climacteric symptoms and serum levels of estradiol, progesterone, follicle-stimulating hormone, and luteinizing hormone. Am J Obstet Gynecol 129:65, 1977

15.   Hutton JD, Jacobs HS, Murray MAF, James VHT: Relation between plasma oestrone and oestradiol and climacteric symptoms. Lancet 1:678, 1978

16.   Heller CG, Farney JP, Myers GP: Development and correlation of menopausal symptoms, vaginal smear and urinary gonadotropin changes following castration in 27 women. J Clin Endocrinol 4:101, 1941

17.   Kupperman HS, Blatt MHG, Wiesbader H, Filler W: Comparative clinical evaluation of estrogenic preparations by menopausal and amenorrhoeal indices. J Clin Endocrinol Metab 13:688, 1953

18.   Newton M, Odom PL: The menopause and its symptoms. South Med J 57:1309, 1964

19.   Serr DM, Rabau E, Mannor S: Correlation of menopausal symptoms with oestrogen deficiency. Clin Trials J 5:91, 1968

20.   Subcommittee of Council of Medical Women's Federation of England: Investigation of menopause in 1000 women. Lancet 1:106, 1933

21.   Wilson RA, Wilson TA: The fate of non-treated postmenopausal women—a plea for the maintenance of adequate estrogen from puberty to the grave. J Am Geriatr Soc 11:347, 1963

22.   Novak ER: Menopause. JAMA 156:575, 1954

23.   van Keep PA: The menopause, a study of the attitudes of women in Belgium, France, Great Britain, Italy and West Germany. Geneva, International Health Foundation, 1970

24.   van Keep PA, Kellerhals J: The aging woman. Front Horm Res 2:160, 1973

25.   Van Look PF, Lothian H, Hunter WM, Michie EA, Baird DT: Hypothalamic-pituitary-ovarian function in perimenopausal women. Clin Endocrinol 7:13, 1977

26.   Treloar AE, Boynton RE, Behn BG, Brown BW: Variability of the human menstrual cycle through reproductive life. Int J Fertil 12:77, 1967

27.   Sherman BM, Korenman SG: Hormonal characteristics of the human menstrual cycle throughout reproductive life. J Clin Invest 55:699, 1975

28.   Utian WH: Use of vaginal smear in assessment of oestrogenic status of oophorectomized females. S Afr J Obstet Gynaecol 8:69, 1970

29.   Lauritzen C: The management of the premenopausal and the postmenopausal patient. Front Horm Res 2:2, 1973

30.   Campbell S: Double-blind psychometric studies on the effects of natural oestrogens in postmenopausal women. In Campbell S (ed): The Management of the Menopause and Postmenopausal Years. Lancaster, MTP Press, 1976

31.   Mulley G, Mitchell JRA, Tattersall RB: Hot flushes after hypophysectomy. Br Med J 2:1062, 1977

32.   Sturdee DW, Wilson KA, Pipili E, Crocker A: Physiological aspects of menopausal hot flush. Br Med J 2:79, 1978

33.   Ginsburg J, Swinhoe J: Physiological aspects of the menopausal hot flush. Br Med J 2:501, 1978

34.   Metz SA, Halter JB, Porte D, Robertson RP: Suppression of plasma catecholamines and flushing by clonidine in man. J Clin Endocrinol Metab 46:83, 1978

35.   Utian WH: Current status of menopause and postmenopausal estrogen therapy. Obstet Gynecol Surv 32:193, 1977

36.   Utian WH: Effect of hysterectomy, oophorectomy and estrogen on libido. Int J Gynaecol Obstet 13:97, 1975

37.   Maoz B, Antonovsky A, Apter A, Wijsenbeek H, Datan N: The perception of menopause in five ethnic groups in Israel. Acta Obstet Gynecol Scand Suppl 65:69, 1977

38.   Maoz B, Antonovsky A, Apter A, et al.: The effect of outside work on the menopausal woman. Maturitas 1:43, 1978

39.   Fedor-Freybergh P, Zador G: Some methodological aspects in the psychosomatic gynaecology. Acta Obstet Gynecol Scand 56:375, 1977

40.   Fedor-Freybergh P: The influence of oestrogens on the well-being and mental performance in climacteric and postmenopausal women. Acta Obstet Gynecol Scand Suppl 64:1, 1977

41.   Derogatis LR, Lipman RS, Covi L: SCL-90—an outpatient psychiatric rating scale—preliminary report. Psychopharmacol Bull 9:13, 1973

42.   Derogatis LR, Lipman RS, Rickels K, Uhlenhuth EH, Covi L: The Hopkins symptom checklist (HSCL): A self-report symptom inventory. Behav Sci 19:1, 1974

43.   Dennerstein L, Burrows GD: A review of studies of the psychological symptoms found at the menopause. Maturitas 1:55, 1978

44.   Brown JRWC, Brown MEC: Psychiatric disorders associated with the menopause. In Beard R (ed): The Menopause. Lancaster, MTP Press, 1976, p 57

45.   Rybo G, Westerberg H: Symptoms in the postmenopause, a population study. Acta Obstet Gynaecol Scand 30:25, 1971

46.   Winokur G: Depression in the menopause. Am J Psychiatry 130:92, 1973

47.   Neugarten BL, Kraines RJ: Menopausal symptoms in women of various ages. Psychosom Med 27:266, 1965

48.   Crawford MP, Hooper D: Menopause, aging and family. Soc Sci Med 7:469, 1975

49.   Ballinger CB: Psychiatric morbidity and the menopause: screening of a general population sample. Br Med J 3:344, 1975

50.   Forman JB: Hormonal vs psychosomatic disturbances of the menopause. Psychosomatics Suppl 9:17, 1978

51.   Hertz DG, Steiner JE, Zuckerman H, Pizanti S: Psychological and physical symptom formation in menopause. Psychother Psychosom 19:47, 1971

52.   Flint M: The menopause, reward or punishment. Psychosomatics 16:161, 1975

53.   van Keep PA, Humphrey M: Psycho-social aspects of the climacteric. In van Keep PA (ed): Consensus on Menopause Research. Lancaster, MTP Press, 1976, p. 5

54.   Utian WH: The Menopause Manual. A Woman's Guide to the Menopause. Lancaster, MTP Press, 1979

55.   Kuhn ME: Sexual myths surrounding the aging. In Oaks, Melchiode, Ficher (eds): Sex and the Life Cycle. New York, Grune and Stratton, 1976, p. 117

56.   Dennerstein L, Wood C, Burrows GDB: Sexual response following hysterectomy and oophorectomy. Obstet Gynecol 49:92, 1977

8

Risks Versus Benefits of Replacement Hormones

Numerous potential benefits have been claimed for postmenopausal replacement of the sex steroid hormones, singly or in combination, in a vast medical literature that ranges from highly scientific to anecdotal. This chapter has three objectives: (1) review the potential benefits of such therapy; (2) evaluate the possible risks; and (3) demonstrate how the risks and benefits of long-term estrogen therapy after menopause can be balanced by the application of general analytic methods. Unnecessary duplication of material already discussed will be avoided by reference to the appropriate chapters.

POTENTIAL BENEFITS

Relief of Symptoms

Certain specific symptoms are estrogen-related and these are more likely to respond to estrogen therapy. Based on the previous discussion, the specific early symptoms are those related to hot flushes and atrophic vaginitis (Chapter 7). In turn, they have been shown to respond to short-term estrogen therapy as tested on single-blind estrogen-placebo cross-over studies,[1,2] double-blind studies,[3,4] in innumerable clinical reports over the years,[5-11] and in most physicians' clinical experience.

It should come as no surprise that nonspecific symptoms have been less successfully treated with estrogen. In this instance, the hormone cannot be blamed; rather, it is mandatory for the clinician to look for the specific indication. Correctly, nonspecific symptoms should be fully investigated for a different pathologic cause.

Late symptoms that result from long-term estrogen deficiency problems are unlikely to be responsive to estrogen replacement unless such therapy has been proven to cure the pathology as well. Backache due to osteoporosis, for example, is unlikely to respond to estrogens for reasons discussed in Chapter 5.

Prevention of Osteoporosis

The prevention of osteoporosis and its complications is one of the most cited indications for long-term estrogen therapy, and is discussed in detail in Chapter 5.

The Mental Tonic Effect

The mental tonic effect described by Utian[12] has been confirmed as an entity that is independent of vasomotor symptoms.[3,4,13] That is, postmenopausal women receiving exogenous estrogen therapy feel better in terms of mental awareness and ability to perform their daily duties, and thus have a generally improved feeling of well-being. A specially devised scoring system for assessment of the general state of mental well-being was applied to 50 oophorectomized women in a prospective estrogen-placebo crossover study. While a definitive placebo response was shown to exist, estrogen proved to be significantly superior to placebo.[12] It is this euphoric effect or general improvement in mental state that probably ac-

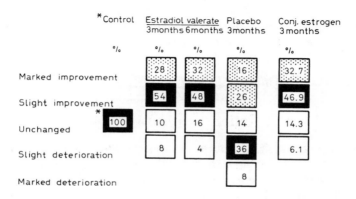

Figure 8-1.   Investigator's measure of mental tonic response to estrogen and placebo therapy in 50 oophorectomized women (From Utian: Front Horm Res 3:74, 1975. Courtesy Karger Publishers.)

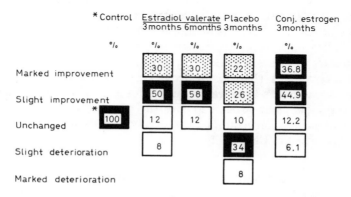

Figure 8-2.   Patient's personal impression of mental tonic response to estrogen and placebo treatment (From Utian: Front Horm Res 3:74, 1975. Courtesy Karger Publishers.)

counts for the reduction in some nonspecific symptoms that are not directly related to estrogen deficiency (Figures 8-1 and 8-2).[1,12]

The ability of exogenously administered estrogen to improve mental state may reflect a pharmacologic effect, rather than reversal of a post-menopausal phenomenon. Nevertheless, it is a distinct benefit and should be recognized as such.

Effect on Skin

While the thickness of the epidermis and the number of mitoses decreases sharply after castration, it has been shown that pathologic deterioration can be prevented or reduced with estrogen therapy.[14] Moreover, a positive effect of 17 α-estradiol has been demonstrated on skin collagen.[14A] There is, therefore, slight evidence that estrogen prevents skin atrophy but further study is necessary (Chapter 4).

Benefits Claimed but Unproven

Many other potential benefits of long-term estrogen replacement have been claimed, but are unproven. A few are worthy of discussion.

PREVENTION OF AGING   Claims have been made for estrogen in the prevention of aging.[15] In this context "aging" is a nebulous term that needs definition and quantification. If reduced bone loss or deceleration of skin atrophy are components of prevention of aging, then the claim may be true. Otherwise there is as yet no satisfactory study that differentiates estrogen effect from the concurrent processes in a general aging population over a sufficient period of time and in a large enough study group. Until some preliminary evidence is forthcoming, the case must be considered unproven. Estrogen, moreover, could only be one small factor out of many that relate to the aging process.

PREVENTION OF CORONARY HEART DISEASE   The apparent protective effect of the ovary in development of atherosclerosis and coronary heart disease (Chapter 6) has led to claims that long-term estrogen therapy may reduce the incidence of coronary heart disease. Such claims have not held true.

IMPROVEMENT IN LIBIDO   Unsubstantiated claims have also been made for the use of estrogen in improving libido after menopause. Decreased libido due to vaginal atrophy (that is, the patient who "wants" but "can't") will respond to local effects of estrogen on the vaginal epithelium.[16] Estrogen replacement, in the absence of local vaginal problems, has been shown to be of no benefit in the treatment of decreased or absent libido.[17,18]

RELIEF OF MINOR PSYCHIATRIC SYMPTOMS   The actual status of estrogens for the treatment of minor psychiatric symptoms (e.g., minor depression, irritability, insomnia) is less clear. Initially, there were an extraordinarily wide number of claims for beneficial effects of estrogens on psychological changes, but few have held up to scrutiny.[19-22] Many investigators were unable to differentiate estrogen effects on psychological symptoms from placebo responses.[1,23,24]

Kantor and co-workers reported estrogens to delay the "psychologic deterioration" that apparently occurs in untreated older women.[25,26] Fedor-Freybergh confirmed the ability of estrogen to slow down the natural deterioration of some perceptual, attentional, and memory processes.[13] Thomson and Oswald reported estrogens to increase rapid eye movement sleep, that is, to be of possible value in the postmenopausal patient complaining of insomnia.[24]

The difficulty in reaching any significant conclusion as to a precise role for estrogens in relief of minor psychiatric symptoms could be blamed on a "symptom-snowball" effect. That is, the beneficial effect of estrogens on hot flushes reduces night sweats and this enhances the ability to sleep, which in turn has a positive influence on mood, which increases the ability to concentrate, and so forth. There is a need for a randomized, controlled, prospective, double-blind study of the effects of estrogens in postmenopausal women without hot flushes for their effect on these minor symptoms.[4] In the interim, the mental tonic effect aside, the case for estrogens must be considered as possible, but unproven (Chapter 7).

POTENTIAL RISKS

The possible risks of estrogen therapy, in general, have been as poorly defined as the potential benefits. The reason for this is not a want of trying, but rather is due to the tremendous problems involved in analyzing risk. It is extremely difficult to assess the risk attributable to one factor like estrogen without considering the synergistic effects of other health risk factors such as smoking, obesity, and hypertension, and possible other coincidental factors which are not as easily identified. For example, contraceptive pill users who are nonsmokers appear to be at lower risk of heart disease mortality than pill users who do smoke cigarettes.[27] Does the same apply to pure estrogen? Moreover, these synergistic influences vary in different countries and within different socioeconomic groups in a given country. It is not always possible to determine in many studies whether such potential synergistic effects have been considered.

Despite the above limitations, some risks to long-term estrogen usage have become obvious and merit consideration.[28,29]

Postmenopausal Bleeding

This is a real disadvantage of postmenopausal estrogen therapy. The incidence will vary depending on prescribing practices, drug selection, and dosage, and on patient response. Older women strongly associate bleeding after menopause with cancer, and they should be spared this unnecessary cause for anxiety. Differentiation is occasionally made between "on-pill" bleeding and "between-pill" bleeding. In either event, endometrial biopsy and even dilation and curettage is usually indicated, particulary as a regular bleeding response to estrogen is no guarantee of a healthy endometrium.[30]

Endometrial response to circulating estrogens and progesterone were fully discussed in Chapter 4. Unopposed estrogen stimulation may lead to excessive proliferation, or hyperplasia, the clinical management of which will be reviewed in Chapter 10, and details of the pathogenesis described in the section on uterine cancer below.

Unnecessary Surgery

estrogen therapy → postmenopausal bleeding → hysterectomy !!

The increased incidence of postmenopausal bleeding may directly affect the incidence of diagnostic curettage and hysterectomy. For instance, the rate of hysterectomy in the United States is said to have increased from 602/100,000 in 1970 to 727/100,000 in 1975.[31,32] What is not known is the influence, if any, of estrogen therapy on this increase. There is an urgent need for these statistics.

Uterine Cancer

Until late 1975, little heed was given to the potential for uterine cancer, although warnings about possible estrogen risk had appeared in early reviews.[33] Then a series of papers appeared which linked estrogen usage with the possibility of an increased risk of uterine cancer.[34-36] Thereby commenced a debate which became, at times, extremely acrimonious and has been reflected in an extraordinarily large literature. Many detailed reviews of the debate,[31,37-39] and of the postulations for the theoretical basis for such an increase in the risk[40-43] have appeared in print. Following the publication of further reports with relative risk ratios similar to those in the original papers,[44-48B] it is now possible to apply some perspective to the situation.

What is the risk? How large?

ENDOMETRIAL HYPERPLASIA   Continuous unopposed estrogen stimulation from both endogenous and exogenous sources can cause hyperplasia of the endometrium. The changes range from a simple hyperplasia to lesions which are difficult to differentiate from invasive adenocarcinoma of the endometrium.[49,50]

Description of these lesions has unfortunately been plagued by a variable terminology. Wentz has termed the alterations of greatest clinical interest the "dysplastic endometrial lesions." These include adenomatous hyperplasia, atypical hyperplasia, and adenocarcinoma *in situ*.[51] Each of these lesions has a distinct histologic appearance, although transitions between them are frequent. The definitive histological characteristics of these three conditions have been very lucidly described and illustrated by Vellios.[52,53]

The relative frequency of the various hyperplasias was evaluated by Wentz, who reported an increased frequency of these conditions in 1974.[51] Sturdee et al. assessed the contributions of various regimens of estrogen therapy to variable bleeding patterns and endometrial histology.[30] Cyclical unopposed oral estrogen treatment was associated with a 12 percent incidence of endometrial hyperplasia. Whitehead suggested that endometrial hyperplasia after unopposed cyclic estrogens was dose-dependent. He reported a 32 percent incidence of cystic glandular and atypical hyperplasia with high-dose estrogens, and a 16 percent incidence with lower doses of estrogen.[49] The varying endometrial response to different estrogens has been reviewed by Myhre.[50]

Siiteri et al. postulated a specific effect of estrone, different from estradiol, on the endometrial target cells.[54] This so-called "estrone hypothesis" postulated that unopposed exposure of target tissues to estrone may be a causal factor in the development of cancer. This theory has not held up to detailed scrutiny. Tseng and Gurpide have shown *in vitro* that the estrogen tightly bound to nuclei is not estrone, but estradiol, even when estrone is the only estrogen supplied to human endometrium.[55] Thijssen and co-workers have presented *in vivo* evidence to confirm this, specifically a consistently higher estradiol/estrone ratio in uterine tissue compared to peripheral plasma.[56]

The controversy surrounding the dysplastic endometrial lesions relates to the question of whether they are premalignant lesions that can progress to invasive endometrial carcinoma. Wentz has listed some of the problems in assessing the true precancerous potential of these lesions, including (1) the variable histologic criteria used for diagnosis, (2) the fact that involvement can be diffuse or focal, (3) the role of concurrent exogenous hormone therapy, (4) the regressive character of lesions after curettage, (5) coexistence with invasive adenocarcinoma, and (6) frequent failure to define the pre- or postmenopausal state of the patient.[51] Nonetheless, the dysplastic endometrial lesions are suspected by many authorities to precede and coexist with endometrial cancer.[51-53,57,58]

The treatment of these lesions depends upon numerous variables, including the age and parity of the patient, her reproductive history, and the specific histologic characteristics. Many consider that the first line of treatment in the perimenopausal patient should be progestogen therapy,[51,53,59] a subject discussed further in Chapters 9 and 10. Sturdee et al. showed that the 12 percent incidence of endometrial hyperplasia on continuous unopposed oral estrogen therapy could be reduced to 8 percent with a 5-day course of progestogen, and to 0 percent if the progestogen was given for 10 days.[30] It has also been suggested that use of progestogens will not only convert hyperplastic to normal endometrium, but that these drugs will prevent the progression of the endometrial dysplasias to invasive cancer.[30,49,59,60]

ESTROGENS AND ENDOMETRIAL CANCER

The annual risk of development of endometrial cancer in untreated women after the menopause with an intact uterus is usually accepted as being about one in every thousand. The general consensus of the studies linking long-term estrogen therapy to endometrial cancer is that the annual cancer risk will be increased to between four and eight cases per thousand.[34-36, 44-47,61] In particular, the following factors seem to enhance the relationship between estrogen and cancer:

1. An increase in duration of therapy to more than three years doubles the risk ratio from 4.6 to 9.2.[45,61]
2. The type of drug may be of importance, nonsteroidal estrogens and estrone preparations possibly being of greater risk.[44,61] In fairness, however, these were also the most available and frequently used estrogens, and this aspect needs further clarification.
3. The risk increases with higher dosage of estrogen.[45,46,61]
4. Continuous unopposed estrogen administration is a greater risk factor than cycled therapy in the risk production.[45,46] Two recent studies call this statement into question, and at this time the matter remains unresolved.[48A,B]

Two important issues need to be raised. First, the question as to whether estrogen is a carcinogen or a cocarcinogen is not the pertinent one. The maximal definable risk is the pertinent issue. That is, the question is not whether estrogen causes cancer, within present knowledge, but rather what is the worst possible risk that may be entailed if estrogen does cause cancer. The answer, as stated above, appears to lie between an extra four to eight cases per year per one thousand women treated. This would seem to be true despite earlier case-control studies which reported no increased risk[62,63] and criticisms of the analytic methods for case control studies[64] which, in turn, have stimulated counter-criticisms.[65]

Second, if such an increased relationship does exist, and the evidence now appears strong, then what factors could explain this increased risk and are such factors avoidable? Again, the consensus of the above studies appears to indicate that the risk is maximized in unselected women placed on continuous high dosages of estrogen over a long period of time.

Certain individuals do appear to be at increased risk for endometrial cancer.[43,66] Moreover, a continuous high-estrogen status is nonphysiologic.[40] It is possible that lower doses of selected estrogen given cyclically with added progestogen in some instances,[30,31,48B,60,67] to a patient without known cancer-risk factors and who is adequately and regularly observed,[28,60] may result in an incidence of carcinoma similar to that of nontreated patients. There is theoretical reason to expect this but little proof, and the final answer will have to await the reports of various avenues of research currently in progress.

Breast Cancer

The relationship between estrogen therapy and the risk for development of breast cancer is more clouded. A possible marginal increase in breast carcinoma in estrogen-treated patients has been reported[68] but has not been confirmed.[69,70] At worst, the relative risk appears to be increased by a factor of 1.3 at 12 years of estrogen therapy and by a factor of 2 after 15 years of usage.[68]

Once again, as with estrogens and endometrial cancer, the risk appears to be related to the continuous long-term use of relatively high dosages of estrogens. There is, as yet, no evidence as to whether cyclical low-dose estrogen with added progestogen will affect the development of breast cancer. Experience from use of the oral contraceptive is reassuring in this respect. None of the published retrospective studies or prospective studies have indicated any overall relationship between oral contraceptive use and breast cancer.[29]

Mammography has been of considerable value in evaluating the breast. However, estrogen therapy after menopause can produce changes in the breast demonstrable as cystic or dysplastic by mammography.[71] These changes regress on cessation of therapy and it has therefore been suggested that such therapy be discontinued before mammography so that clinical and radiologic evaluation can be enhanced.[71]

Deep Vein Thrombosis and Thromboembolism

It is nearly a quarter of a century since a small group of women in Puerto Rico were rendered temporarily infertile by a daily dose of an estrogen-progestogen mixture. One of the most worrisome of the untoward consequences of this therapy has been the effect on the blood clotting mechanism with the risk of thromboembolic phenomena and death. Despite the numerous investigations into this problem, there are still many unexplained aspects and inevitable areas of disagreement.

Most authorities agree that the oral contraceptive is associated with a definite risk of venous thrombosis, thromboembolism, and possible death.[72,73] Furthermore, it is also generally accepted that this risk is causally related, and not simply the initiation of an inherent predisposition to thrombosis.[74] But some dissension does exist and this relationship has been questioned.[75,76]

It is not surprising, therefore, that far more disagreement exists on the question of a relationship between postmenopausal estrogen usage and thromboembolic phenomena. Unlike the information on oral contraceptive usage, there are no good statistics for deep venous thrombosis and thromboembolism on estrogen therapy when given alone.

The question of thromboembolic risk is extremely important. The concept of long-term estrogen replacement following menopause implies that such drug usage will reduce certain risk factors such as the development of osteoporosis. The value would be negated were one risk factor to be replaced by another; the same argument, of course, holds true for endometrial cancer. Moreover, it would appear that the patients to receive postmenopausal estrogens would be at higher risk for development of thromboembolism, often being obese, hypertensive, cigarette smokers, and mostly over the age of 50.

There is preliminary evidence to suggest that the risk of thromboembolism may be increased in postmenopausal estrogen users compared to nonusers. The risk appears to be increased in users of synthetic unconjugated steroids (ethinyl-estradiol and mestranol)[77] as compared to users of conjugated equine estrogen,[78,79] estradiol valerate, or estriol succinate.[80] The latter finding does seem to be a specific drug-related response, rather than a dose-related effect, in that all the estrogens thus far incriminated in clinical reports as potential thrombogenics are unnatural compounds with an alkylated side chain which renders their metabolism and inactivation slow and inefficient (Chapter 9). It is possible that the use of natural estrogens such as estradiol, estrone or estriol would avoid the problem of thrombosis altogether.

Several authors have investigated the effects of various estrogens on coagulation factors, thus far with conflicting results. Coope and co-workers found natural and synthetic estrogens to raise levels of factors VII and X and to accelerate the prothrombin time,[81] that is, to accelerate blood-clotting values. In a follow-up study, the same group of investigators demonstrated thrombin-induced platelet aggregation to be significantly accelerated after 18 months conjugated estrogen treatment.[82] This suggested a widening spectrum of effect. Stangel et al., confirmed this with a report of a 289 percent increase in the hypercoagulability of the blood of women treated with conjugated estrogens.[83]

On the other hand, Bolton et al. found neither conjugated equine estrogen nor ethinyl estradiol to affect certain hemostasis-related factors.[78] Notelovitz and Greig,[79] from an assessment of several coagulation factors, confirmed that conjugated estrogens, taken for one year, do not produce a hypercoagulable state. Toy and co-workers compared ethinyl estradiol to estriol succinate in a randomized cross-over study.[80] While no significant change in hemostatic function was observed with estriol succinate, the ethinyl estradiol casued shortening of the prothrombin time and an in-increase in the plasma concentration of factor VII and plasminogen. It should also be noted that of all the estrogens, only ethinyl-estradiol seems to have any significant effect on platelet electrophoretic behavior.[84] Notelovitz and Greig reported a depressant effect of conjugated estrogens on the platelet count, but were unable to explain the finding.[79]

The significance of the reported effects of different estrogens on various coagulation-related factors in clinical terms is far from clear. The early promise that naturally occurring estrogens may be safer than synthetic estrogens is inconclusive but encouraging. Until the situation is clarified, it would appear necessary to avoid estrogen usage in patients with preexisting risk factors for thromboembolism, particularly a previous history of deep venous thrombosis or severe varicosities, obesity, hypertension, diabetes, and heavy smoking. It is likely that postmenopausal estrogen replacement will carry a clinical risk of thromboembolism greater than that of the contraceptive pill in view of the type of population to receive such therapy. Large epidemiologic, clinical, and laboratory-based studies are urgently needed.

The reassuring factor, thus far, has been the failure to find a statistically significant association between current regular use of estrogen and nonfatal acute myocardial infarction or stroke.[85]

Increase in Blood Pressure

The relationship between estrogen, endogenous and exogenous, and blood pressure is unclear.[86] Arterial blood pressure tends to increase with age until late in life. Young women have blood pressure levels similar to young men. The increase with age in women, however, is more rapid, and after middle age their levels exceed those of males.[87,88]

[handwritten note at top: What's the difference in effect between ↑ diastolic BP? ↑ systolic BP?]

Menopause, and supposedly estrogen deficiency, has been a natural target of suspicion for the sexual difference in blood pressure. Data from the United States Health Examination Survey of Adults confirm that women whose menstrual periods had stopped had higher levels of diastolic blood pressure, but not systolic blood pressure, than premenopausal women. The blood pressure levels were not related to type of menopause (spontaneous vs. operative) or time interval since menopause. Although these results were suggestive that menopause precedes the rise in diastolic blood pressure, it was not possible to be certain of the temporal sequence of events.[89]

Von Eiff attempted to explain the increase in blood pressure after menopause as being due to the loss of a premenopausal protective effect of estrogen. His studies suggest that both exogenous and endogenous estrogens play a role in protecting premenopausal women from essential hypertension.[90]

Unfortunately, a paradox seems to exist. Use of the oral contraceptive is associated with a slight, but usually reversible, rise in the mean blood pressure. Fisch and Frank reported the contraceptive-induced blood pressure elevation to be about 5-6 mm Hg systolic and 1-2 mm diastolic, a slight but statistically significant finding.[91] Others have reported similar findings.[92] Moreover, the Royal College of General Practitioners' prospective study on 46,000 women reported that oral contraceptive users were 2 to 2.5 times more likely to develop hypertension than nonusers.[93]

Notelovitz found conjugated estrogens to increase the mean systolic and diastolic blood pressures when administered to postmenopausal women, but only the diastolic was significantly elevated.[94] Spellacy and Birk found oral contraceptives with synthetic estrogens to induce blood pressure elevations, but not conjugated estrogens.[95] Pallas et al. could discern no effect of conjugated estrogens on the blood pressure when corrected for age and relative weight of 575 women on no medication compared to that of 82 on conjugated estrogen.[96] Erkkola et al. could find no effects of estriol succinate on the renin-aldosterone system or on the bodyweight.[97]

The paradox thus appears to be at an impasse. A study by Utian is therefore of interest in that no significant differences in diastolic blood pressure were demonstrated on either estradiol valerate or conjugated estrogen therapy when compared group to group. Nonetheless, the conjugated estrogen treatment group was associated with extreme elevations of the diastolic blood pressure in 2 out of 49 patients.[86]

The lack of a general association of estrogens with any significant elevation of diastolic blood pressure is reassuring. No apparent reason, therefore, exists for withholding estrogen therapy on this basis alone. Nevertheless, observation that some postmenopausal women have an idiosyncratic response to conjugated estrogens with blood pressure elevations is worthy of emphasis.[86,94] In view of the potential adverse effects of such a blood pressure increase, all women on long-term estrogen treatment should have blood pressure readings taken every 6 months as part of their routine medical follow-up examination.

Gallstones   *up 2.5 times.*

The incidence of gallstones, or certainly that of gallstones requiring surgical treatment, has been reported to be increased by a factor of 2.5 in women taking estrogens after menopause.[70] This may be related to the increase in triglycerides reported for estrogen therapy (Chapter 6).[78,92] Whatever the etiology, the relationship appears real. In gross figures, the incidence rate of gallbladder disease requiring surgical treatment increases from 87/100,000 per year in healthy women aged 45 to 49 not on estrogens to 218/100,000 for estrogen users. This is a relative risk of 2.5 times that of a control group.[70]

Surgically corrected gallstones are increased in frequency in women on the oral contraceptive.[73] Pregnancy or estrogen therapy results in cholestasis.[98] Moreover, in animals exposed to estrogen the secretion of bile salts is reduced in a dose-dependent manner.[99]

It is interesting to speculate that the as yet incompletely elucidated effects of estrogens on lipid and lipoprotein metabolism may hold the key to explaining the pathogenesis of gallstones.

Changes in Glucose Tolerance

A number of factors play a confounding role in all studies on carbohydrate metabolism. These include population characteristics, dietary and socioeconomic factors, and genetic predisposition.[100] There is therefore a large body of profoundly contradictory data and a wide diversity of opinion.[100-103] Moreover, the complexities of the problem are further increased by the type and dosage of estrogen and progestogen used and their interactions at various biologic levels.[100,104,105] Finally, most studies on estrogens and progestogens have been applied to oral contraceptive populations and very few in relation to use after menopause.

In general, the effect of exogenous estrogens on glucose tolerance of postmenopausal women has been reassuring. Few significant changes have been found in either the fasting glucose values, glucose tolerance curves, or on plasma insulin levels.[103,105-107] However, some idiosyncratic responses may occur.[106,107]

Notelovitz felt that conjugated estrogens could impair glucose tolerance in a small percentage of patients.[106,107] Thom et al., however, did not find conjugated equine estrogen or estradiol valerate to impair glucose tolerance,[105] and recently Goldzieher and co-workers, in an extremely well-controlled study, were unable to show any adverse effect of ethinyl estradiol or mestranol on carbohydrate metabolism.[100] Nor were they able to demonstrate any effect of added progestogen compounds on estrogen-treated women.[100] Nonetheless, Spellacy et al. believe that estrogen-progestogen combinations may have a synergistic effect and impair glucose tolerance,[103] and, indeed, Thom et al. did show a significant deterioration of carbohydrate tolerance in patients on combinations of ethinyl-estradiol or mestranol with progestogens.[106]

Spellacy et al. reported a significant increase in bodyweight in patients on estrogen therapy.[103] This finding was not confirmed by Utian,[86] nor by McKay et al. who actually found a decrease in weight on estrogen therapy.[88]

Goldzieher has emphasized that glucose intolerance and diabetes mellitus are not the same thing, and that it is inappropriate to infer that any steroid-induced changes carry with them the long-term hazards associated with diabetes mellitus.[100,108]

It can be concluded at this time that correct estrogen usage does not generally result in significant or prolonged alterations in glucose tolerance. However, risk factors such as a family history of diabetes, suggestive obstetric history of potential diabetes, and obesity should be carefully evaluated before prescribing estrogens. Diabetes does not of itself stand as an absolute contraindication to estrogen treatment. It is recommended that a two-hour post-glucose blood level be measured once a year in all patients, diabetic or not, on long-term estrogen therapy.

BALANCING THE RISKS AND BENEFITS

It is obvious that the tradeoff between risks and benefits, or risk: benefit ratio, is finely balanced.* This leads to difficulty in decision-making as to whether estrogen should be administered or not. There are two methods of addressing this problem. The first is to apply what may be termed the *minimax concept.*[109] That is, aim to minimize the risks and maximize the benefits. This necessitates giving due care to factors such

*This section is freely abstracted from a contribution to an International Health Foundation Workshop on The Risks and Benefits of Estrogen Therapy (Utian: Application of cost-effectiveness analysis to postmenopausal estrogen therapy. Front Horm Res 5:26, 1978, courtesy of Karger Publishers). Acknowledgement is also made to Weinstein and Stason: Foundations of cost-effectiveness analysis for health and medical practices. N Engl J Med 296:716, 1977, courtesy of New England Journal of Medicine.

as detailed clinical evaluation so that patients with risk factors do not receive therapy, specific selection of drug, therapeutic regime, added progestogen, detailed follow up, and so forth.

The second approach is to attempt a precise measurement of risk and benefit. An attempt at evaluation of the risk-benefit ratio of the long-term effects of pure estrogens highlights the fact that, compared to the great many carefully designed large-scale epidemiologic studies on the health consequences of oral contraceptive use, no comparable body of data is available for pure estrogen. Despite this lack, it is possible to subject these risks and benefits, and their potential costs, to some form of mathematical evaluation and analysis and to come out with some answer or direction.[109-111]

General Analytic Approaches

Various measures have been designed that can help guide present and future decision making for systematic analysis.[111,112] For example, answers may be needed to problems in allocation of limited health care resources or as aids to health care decision makers in planning new facilities. As mentioned, the balancing of benefits of estrogen therapy against potential risks is a subject in need of such analysis. The answer we seek in this instance should help physicians decide whether such therapy should be given or not.

To be of value, any form of analysis must be comprehensive and broadly applicable. This necessitates the availability of the best current information on both the efficacy of therapy and its costs, as well as the possible risks and their respective costs. Unfortunately, the available data base on the effectiveness of most clinical procedures, estrogen therapy and menopause included, is distressingly limited. This is not reason to despair. There is, for example, a tendency among physicians and consumers to demand exact scientific proof. Although this is commendable and desirable it does not detract from the above principle. In point of fact, until accurate information is obtained, current analysis and decision making must depend upon the best available current evidence. Nonetheless, any form of analysis should be structured to incorporate new data as it becomes available and even to suggest areas in need of future research to resolve critical uncertainties.[111]

An ideal measure of the effectiveness of a clinical practice needs to be outcome-oriented, with length and quality of life as the ultimate measures. Inevitably, when risks and benefits of a particular form of therapy are being evaluated, which in turn involve possible tradeoffs between longevity and quality of life, subjective values have to be involved.

Another area that needs incorporation into any effective analysis is the balance between present and future health benefits and costs. Estrogen therapy, for example, can be considered as a preventive program in which the costs are immediate and ongoing, but the health benefits and risks may be in the future.

Specific Analytic Approaches

Cost-benefit analysis[112] and cost-effectiveness analysis[111] are two different analytic approaches to assessment of health practices.

COST-BENEFIT ANALYSIS   Values all outcomes in economic (e.g. dollar) terms. This requires that human lives and quality of life be valued in dollars. Once the benefits and costs have been reduced to dollar values, the decision whether to administer a form of therapy, in theory at least, is simplified.

COST-EFFECTIVENESS ANALYSIS   In this instance priority is placed on alternate expenditures without requiring that the dollar value of life and health be assessed.[111] Health effectiveness is measured in quality-adjusted life years or QALY because it incorporates changes in survival and morbidity in a single measure that reflects tradeoffs between them. This will be further explained below. Health care costs are measured in dollars. The measure of cost-effectiveness then becomes a ratio of the cost in dollars to net health effectiveness measured in QALY. Thus the lower the ratio, the better the result.

Net Health Care Costs   There are various ways to measure the cost of medical care. Direct (therapeutic) costs include payment for service by doctors, hospitals, laboratories, pharmacy, etc. Use of indirect costs is a more comprehensive measure that takes into account the impact of illness, premature death, or disability on the economy. Being broader in concept, it is less easy to define.

Preventive costs involve the costs of a prophylaxis program which includes drugs, dispensing, education, physician time, etc. Savings on such a program can be calculated by deducting the actual preventive costs from the hypothetical costs of treating the disease in the absence of a prophylactic program. This difference could also be termed avoidable costs.

The following formula for calculation of health costs, modified from Weinstein and Stason,[111] takes all of the above factors, excluding indirect costs, into account:

$$\Delta C = \Delta C_{RX} + \Delta C_{SE} - \Delta C_{BENEF} + \Delta C_{RX\Delta LE}$$

where ΔC = net health care costs (H.C.C.); C_{RX} = all direct H.C.C. (drugs, physician, etc.); ΔC_{SE} = all H.C.C. due to side-effects of treatment; ΔC_{BENEF} = savings in H.C.C. due to disease prevention; and $\Delta C_{RX\Delta LE}$ = H.C.C. of diseases that would not have occurred if patient did not receive treatment.

Net Health Effectiveness   The measure of improvement or loss in quality of life is a controversial area. A weighting scheme or health status index (λS)[110,111] assigns a numerical weight (P) between zero and one to differentiate full health from varying degrees of disability or discomfort. The greater the number the worse the disability, i.e., 0.0 is virtually no disability and 1.0 would imply a patient condition tantamount to being dead, i.e., the probability (P) for death is 1.0. The health status index (λS) is then calculated as 1-P.

The following example demonstrates the use of the Health Status Index to quantify the situation for a potential risk like uterine cancer:

	Morbidity	P
A =	Early cancer removed; no disability	0.05
B =	Surgery plus radiotherapy; no disability	0.15
C =	Vaginal stenosis and pain	0.35
D =	Severe pain, recurrence	0.88
E =	Secondary disease	1.0

$$\lambda S = 1\text{-}P$$
$$\text{and } \lambda S \times \text{Years} = \Delta Y_{CANCER} \; in \; \text{QALY}$$

The potential benefit for prevention of osteoporosis is:

	Morbidity	P
A =	Radiologic osteoporosis; no disability	0.1
B =	Occasional discomfort on exertion	0.35
C =	Fractured wrist	0.55
D =	Femoral neck or vertebral compression fracture	0.85
E =	Totally bedridden, disabled, intractable pain	1.0

$$\lambda S = 1\text{-}P$$
$$\text{and } \lambda S \times \text{Years} = \Delta Y_{OSTEO} \; in \; \text{QALY}$$

The number of years spent (YS) at this health status is multiplied by λS to yield the number of quality adjusted life years (QALY). This can be considered to be equivalent to the number of years spent in full health. The calculation is thus as follows:

$$\lambda S \times YS = \Delta Y_{BENEF} \; or \; \Delta Y_{SE} \; in \; QALY$$

where λS = H.S.I. or disability weight = 1-P, if P = probability of death; YS = years at health status; ΔY_{BENEF} = net health effectiveness; ΔY_{SE} = net health loss; and QALY = quality-adjusted life-years.

The overall measure of improvement or loss in quality of life, or net health effectiveness, can be calculated from the following formula, also modified from Weinstein and Stason:[111]

$$\Delta E = \Delta Y + \Delta Y_{BENEF} - \Delta Y_{SE}$$

where ΔE = net health effectiveness in QALY; ΔY = expected number of unadjusted life years; ΔY_{BENEF} = improvement in quality of life years due to reduction in morbidity or prevention thereof; and ΔY_{SE} = loss due to side effects of treatment.

The expected number of unadjusted life years (ΔY) can be derived from life tables. The measure of ΔY_{BENEF} and of ΔY_{SE} are calculated as previously described.

Unfortunately, data is not usually available to make these measures with certainty, a source of criticism of cost-effectiveness analysis. Furthermore, the whole trade-off concept is difficult. Nonetheless, such trade offs in therapeutic measures are made daily by physicians. All that health analysis does is supply a quantification to make the measure explicit.[111]

COST-EFFECTIVENESS ANALYSIS APPLIED TO POSTMENOPAUSAL ESTROGEN THERAPY

Calculation of the cost effectiveness of long-term estrogen therapy after the menopause is dependent upon numerous local factors in various countries and communities and therefore needs independent analysis. The potential advantages and disadvantages have been dealt with in depth above, as have the areas of deficiency in terms of real statistics. It is worthy of reemphasis that cost-effectiveness analysis takes present knowledge as a data base and allows future knowledge to be incorporated. Potential risks and benefits must be evaluated with this in mind.

In a world beset with problems of inflation, disparity of health programs, and variable health needs, it would be more than presumptuous to attempt to advise on the desirability of a general estrogen prophylaxis program and to estimate costs for such a program for any specific region. It is mandatory, of course, that costs be calculated according to the formula already presented, but that local statistics be utilized.

Some limited attempts have been made at such an analysis. For example, Aitken[113] and Dewhurst[114] have independently estimated that the total annual drug bill for Britain would be about £90,000,000 (approximately $183,000,000) if conjugated estrogens were routinely prescribed for prophylaxis. Dewhurst has calculated that the bill for medical services would add a further £65,000,000 ($132,000,000) per year.[114] Aitken in turn calculated that the annual cost of treating femoral neck and Colles' fractures in a stable population of 200,000 people (in which population there would be about 38,000 women over 45) would be about £40,000 ($81,500), or looked at in wider context about £10,000,000 ($21,000,000) for the whole of Britain per year.[113] This would allow £1 ($2.00) per head per annum before the cost of prophylaxis exceeded the likely cost of treating complications of osteoporosis as they arose. Unfortunately, the British figures do not take into account the Health Status Index, that is, the cost to the patient of being in pain or disabled or unable to live an independent existence. Recalculation of the figures with true cost-effectiveness analysis would therefore be of greater value. In Britain, nonetheless, the cost of prevention of osteoporosis clearly far exceeds the cost of treatment of the developed problem.

Greenwald et al.[38] have estimated that 14 percent of American women over the age of 45 now take estrogens, predominantly conjugated estrogen at a cost of $82,777,000, in 1975 shipments for use in the United States. Aitken estimated that general use of conjugated equine estrogens in Britain could cost about £88,500,000 ($180,000,000) whereas cheap synthetics would cost about £2,600,000 ($5,300,000).

It is apparent that controversy exists. Different estrogens do appear to exert different effects. The answer, therefore, in addition to usage of local statistics, is an urgent need for cost-effectiveness analysis to be applied to the use of all the presently available types of estrogen as well.

CONCLUSIONS

Application of specific analytic methods to long-term estrogen therapy is of value in that it forces physicians and health planners to be explicit about the beliefs and values that underlie their decisions. Where points of view differ, the relative trade offs can be compared more directly.

The balance of risks and benefits is dependent upon a number of unanswered questions. At the present time the decision to prescribe long-term estrogen therapy must rest upon a choice between relying on a proper analysis despite the present imperfections, or on no analysis at all. To quote Weinstein and Stason: "The former, in these times of increasingly complex decisions, difficult tradeoffs, and limited resources, is by far the preferred choice."[111]

Until further results are forthcoming, the following attitudes toward practice could be adopted:

1. Short-term estrogen therapy for specific menopausal symptoms (hot flushes and atrophic vaginitis) is fully acceptable.
2. Long-term hormone therapy is justified in young women undergoing premature menopause, provided the due precautions are observed.
3. Long-term therapy cannot yet be recommended for all women after menopause. It is not, however, justifiable to withhold such treatment from a normal informed patient who requests it on an individual basis, provided there are no contraindications (Chapter 9) and the patient agrees to regular checkups (Chapter 10).
4. Certain rules for estrogen usage and patient follow-up exist and must be observed (Chapters 9, 10). In particular, the drug should be administered cyclically or intermittently, and in the lowest effective dose.

Menopause and estrogen therapy are emotional subjects, not only to women but to men and to doctors. It is mandatory to keep an open mind on the subject, as new evidence is bound to accumulate at an accelerating pace in the near future. In the interim, the advantages should be maximized and the disadvantages minimized for each potential patient.

References

1. Utian WH: The true clinical features of postmenopause and oophorectomy and their response to oestrogen therapy. S Afr Med J 46:732, 1972

2. Utian WH: Comparative trial of P1496, a new non-steroidal estrogen analogue. Br Med J 1:579, 1973

3. Campbell S, Whitehead M : Oestrogen therapy and the menopause syndrome. In Greenblatt RB, Studd JWW (eds): Clinics in Obstetrics and Gynecology. Philadelphia, Saunders, 1977, Vol 4, No 1

4. Campbell S: Double blind psychometric studies on the effects of natural estrogens on post-menopausal women. In Campbell S (ed): The Management of the Menopause. Lancaster, MTP Press, 1976, p. 149

5.   Kullander S, Svanberg L: On climacteric symptoms and their treatment with a new non-steroidal estrogen. Int J Gynaecol Obstet 13:277, 1975

6.   Kupperman HS, Wetchler BB, Blatt MHG: Contemporary therapy of the menopausal syndrome. JAMA 171:1627, 1959

7.   Wilson RA, Brevetti RE, Wilson TA: Specific procedures for the elimination of the menopause. West J Surg Obstet Gynecol 71:110, 1963

8.   Lozman H, Barlow AL, Levitt DG: Piperazine estrone sulfate and conjugated estrogens equine in the treatment of the menopausal syndrome. South Med J 64:1143, 1971

9.   Velikay L: The oral treatment of the climacteric syndrome with oestradiol valerate. Wien Klin Wochenschr 80:229, 1968

10.   Dapunt O: The treatment of climacteric symptoms with oestradiol valerate. Med Klin 62:1356, 1967

11.   Tzingounis VA, Aksu MF, Greenblatt RB: Estriol in the management of the menopause. JAMA 239:1638, 1978

12.   Utian WH: The mental tonic effect of oestrogens administered to oophorectomized females. S Afr Med J 46:1079, 1972

13.   Fedor-Freybergh P: The influence of oestrogens on the wellbeing and mental performance in climacteric and postmenopausal women. Acta Obstet Gynecol Scand Suppl 64, 1, 1977

14.   Punnonen R: Effect of castration and peroral estrogen therapy on the skin. Acta Obstet Gynecol Scand Suppl 21, 1, 1972

14A.   Meyer WJ, Henneman DH, Keiser HR, Bartter FC: 17 α-estradiol — separation of estrogen effect on collagen from other clinical and biochemical effects in man. Res Commun Chem Pathol Pharmacol 13:685, 1976

15.   Wilson RA, Wilson TA: The fate of the nontreated postmenopausal woman. A plea for the maintenance of adequate estrogen from puberty to the grave. J Am Geriatr Soc 11:347, 1963

16.   Utian WH: Use of vaginal smear in assessment of oestrogenic status of oophorectomized females. S Afr Med J 44:69, 1970

17.   Utian WH: Effect of hysterectomy, oophorectomy and estrogen therapy on libido. Int J Gynaecol Obstet 13:97, 1975

18.   Dennerstein L, Wood C, Burrows GD: Sexual response following hysterectomy and oophorectomy. Obstet Gynecol 49:92, 1977

19.   Hawkinson LF: The menopausal syndrome. One thousand consecutive patients treated with estrogen. JAMA 111:390, 1938

20.   Ingvarsson G: Hormone treated cases of menopausal psychosis. Acta Psychiatr Scand 26:155, 1951

21.   Cameron WJ: Endocrine therapy in the menopause. Gen Pract 33:110, 1966

22.   Dennerstein L, Burrows GD: A review of studies of the psychological symptoms found at the menopause. Maturitas 1:55, 1978

23. George GCW, Utián WH, Beumont PJV, Beardwood CJ: Effect of exogenous oestrogens on minor psychiatric symptoms in postmenopausal women. S Afr Med J 47:2387, 1973

24. Thomson J, Oswald I: Effect of oestrogen on the sleep, mood, and anxiety of menopausal women. Br Med J 2:1317, 1977

25. Kantor HI, Michael CM, Shore H, Ludvigson HW: Administration of estrogens to older women, a psychometric evaluation. Am J Obstet Gynecol 101:658, 1968

26. Michael CM, Kantor HI, Shore H: Further psychometric evaluation of older women—the effect of estrogen administration. J Gerontol 25:337, 1970

27. Jain AK: Mortality risk associated with the use of oral contraceptives. Stud Fam Plann 8:50, 1977

28. Utian WH: Current status of menopause and postmenopausal estrogen therapy. Obstet Gynecol Surv 32:193, 1977

29. Utian WH: Estrogen replacement in the menopause. In Wynn R (ed): Obstetrics and Gynecology Annual, 1979. New York, Appleton, 1979

30. Sturdee DW, Wade-Evans T, Paterson MEL, Thom M, Studd JWW: Relations between bleeding pattern, endometrial histology, and oestrogen treatment in normal women. Br Med J 1:1575, 1978

31. Kistner RW: Estrogen and endometrial cancer. Obstet Gynecol 48:479, 1976

32. Editorial: Rate of hysterectomy increases. Obstet Gynecol News 12:2, 1977

33. Utian WH: Feminine forever? Current concepts of the menopause. A critical review. S Afr J Obstet Gynaecol 6:7, 1968

34. Smith DC, Prentice R, Thomson DJ, Herrmann W: Association of exogenous estrogen and endometrial carcinoma. N Engl J Med 293:1164, 1975

35. Ziel HK, Finkle WD: Increased risk of endometrial carcinoma among users of conjugated estrogens. N Engl J Med 293:1167, 1975

36. Mack TM, Pike MC, Henderson BE, et al.: Estrogens and endometrial cancer in a retirement community. N Engl J Med 294:1262, 1976

37. Knab DR: Estrogen and endometrial carcinoma. Obstet Gynecol Surv 32:267, 1977

38. Greenwald P, Caputo TA, Wolfgang PE: Endometrial cancer after menopausal use of estrogens. Obstet Gynecol 50:239, 1977

39. Mack TM: Uterine cancer and estrogen therapy. Front Horm Res 5:101, 1978

40. Gurpide E: Hormones and gynecolgic cancer. Cancer 38:503, 1976

41. Hertz R: The estrogen-cancer hypothesis. Cancer 38:534, 1976

42. Siiteri PK, Schwartz BE, MacDonald PC: Estrogen receptors and the estrone hypothesis in relation to breast and endometrial cancer. Gynecol Oncol 2:228, 1974

43.   Klopper A, Farr J: The epidemiology of endometrial cancer. Front Horm Res 5:89, 1978

44.   Hoover R, Fraumeni JF, Everson R, Myers MH: Cancer of the uterine corpus after hormonal treatment for breast cancer. Lancet 1:885, 1976

45.   Gray LA, Christopherson WM, Hoover RN: Estrogens and endometrial cancer. Obstet Gynecol 49:385, 1977

46.   McDonald TW, Annegers JF, O'Fallon WM, et al.: Exogenous estrogen and endometrial carcinoma: case control and incidence study. Am J Obstet Gynecol 127:572, 1977

47.   Gordon J, Reagan JW, Finkle WK, Ziel HK: Estrogen and endometrial carcinoma. An independent pathology review supporting original risk estimate. N Engl J Med 297:570, 1977

48.   Antunes CMF, Stolley PD, Rosenshein NB, et al.: Endometrial cancer and estrogen use. Report of a large case-control study. N Engl J Med 300:9, 1979

48A.   Jick H, Watkins RN, Hunter JR et al.: Replacement estrogens and endometrial cancer. N Engl J Med 300:218, 1979

48B.   Hammond CB, Jelovsek FR, Lee KL et al.: Effects of long-term estrogen replacement therapy. II Neoplasia. Am J Obstet Gynecol 133:537, 1979

49.   Whitehead MI: The effects of oestrogens and progestogens on the postmenopausal endometrium. Maturitas 1:87, 1978

50.   Myhre E: Endometrial response to different estrogens. Front Horm Res 5:126, 1978

51.   Wentz WB: Progestin therapy in endometrial hyperplasia. Gynecol Oncol 2:362, 1974

52.   Vellios F: Endometrial hyperplasias, precursors of endometrial carcinoma. In Sommers C (ed): Pathology Annual. New York, Appleton, 1972, p. 201

53.   Vellios F: Endometrial hyperplasia and carcinoma in situ. Gynecol Oncol 2:152, 1974

54.   Siiteri PK, Schwartz B, MacDonald PC: Estrogen receptors and the estrone hypothesis in relation to endometrial and breast cancer. Gynecol Oncol 2:228, 1974

55.   Tseng L, Gurpide E: Effect of estrone and progesterone on the nuclear uptake of estradiol by slices of endometrium. Endocrinology 93:245, 1973

56.   Thijssen JHH, Wiegerinek MAHM, Mulder G, Poortman J: On the biological activity of estrone in vivo. Front Horm Res 5:220, 1978

57.   Novak ER, Woodruff JD: Novaks Gynecologic and Obstetric Pathology, 7th ed. Philadelphia, Saunders, 1970

58.   Gusberg SB, Kaplan AL: Precursors of corpus cancer. IV. Adenomatous hyperplasia as stage O carcinoma of the endometrium. Am J Obstet Gynecol 87:662, 1963

59.   Gambrell RH, Castaneda TA, Ricci CA: Management of postmenopausal bleeding to prevent endometrial cancer. Maturitas 1:99, 1978

60.   Gambrell RD: The prevention of endometrial cancer in postmenopausal women with progestogens. Maturitas 1:107, 1978

61.   Ziel HK, Finkle WD: Association of estrone with the development of endometrial carcinoma. Am J Obstet Gynecol 124:735, 1976

62.   Dunn LF, Bradbury JT: Endocrine factors in endometrial carcinoma, a preliminary report. Am J Obstet Gynecol 97:465, 1967

63.   Pacheco JC, Kempers RD: Etiology of postmenopausal bleeding. Obstet Gynecol 32:40, 1968

64.   Horwitz RI, Feinstein AR: Alternative analytic methods for case-control studies of estrogen and endometrial cancer. N Engl J Med 299:1089, 1978

65.   Hutchison GB, Rothman KF: Correcting a bias? N Engl J Med 299:1129, 1978

66.   Gusberg SB: The individual at high-risk for endometrial cancer. Am J Obstet Gynecol 126:535, 1976

67.   Hsueh AJW, Peck EJ, Clark JH: Control of uterine estrogen receptor levels by progesterone. Endocrinology 98:438, 1976

68.   Hoover R, Gray LA, Cole P, MacMahon B: Menopausal estrogens and breast cancer. N Engl J Med 295:401, 1976

69.   Burch JC, Byrd BF, Vaughn WK: The effect of long-term estrogen on hysterectomized women. Am J Obstet Gynecol 118:778, 1974

70.   Boston Collaborative Drug Surveillance Program: surgically confirmed gallbladder disease, venous thromboembolism and breast tumors in relation to postmenopausal estrogen therapy. N Engl J Med 290:15, 1974

71.   Peck DR, Lowman RM: Estrogen and the postmenopausal breast. Mammographic considerations. JAMA 240:1733, 1978

72.   Vessey MP, Doll R: Investigation of the relationship between the use of oral contraceptives and thromboembolic disease. Br Med J 2:199, 1968

73.   Boston Collaborative Drug Surveillance Program: Oral contraceptives and venous thromboembolic disease, surgically confirmed gallbladder disease, and breast tumors. Lancet 1:1399, 1973

74.   Badaracco MA, Vessey MP: Recurrence of venous thromboembolic disease and use of oral contraceptives. Br Med J 1:215, 1974

75.   Drill VA: Oral contraceptives and thromboembolic disease. I. Prospective and retrospective studies. JAMA 219:583, 1972

76.   Drill VA, Calhoun DW: Oral contraceptives and thromboembolic disease. II. Estrogen content of oral contraceptives. JAMA 219:593, 1972

77.   Gow D, MacGillivray I: Metabolic, hormonal and vascular changes after synthetic oestrogen therapy in oophorectomized women. Br Med J 1:73, 1971

78.   Bolton CH, Ellwood M, Hartog M, et al.: Comparison of the effects of ethinyl estradiol and conjugated equine estrogens in oophorectomized women. Clin Endocrinol 4:131, 1975

79.   Notelovitz M, Greig HBW: The effect of natural oestrogens on coagulation. S Afr Med J 49:101, 1975

80.   Toy JL, Davies JA, Hancock KW, McNicol GP: The comparative effects of a synthetic and a natural oestrogen on the haemostatic mechanism in patients with primary amenorrhea. Br J Obstet Gynaecol 85:359, 1978

81.   Coope J, Thompson JM, Poller L: Effects of natural oestrogen replacement therapy on menopausal symptoms and blood clotting. Br Med J 4:139, 1975

82.   Poller L, Thomson JM, Coope J: Conjugated equine estrogens and blood clotting — a follow-up report. Br Med J 1:935, 1977

83.   Stangel JJ, Innerfield J, Reyniak V, Stone ML: The effect of conjugated estrogens on coagulability in menopausal women. Obstet Gynecol 49:314, 1977

84.   Elkeles RS, Hampton JR, Mitchell JRA: Effect of oestrogens on human platelet behavior. Lancet 2:315, 1968

85.   Rosenberg L, Armstrong B, Jick H: Myocardial infarction and estrogen therapy in postmenopausal women. N Engl J Med 294:1256, 1976

86.   Utian WH: Effect of postmenopausal estrogen therapy on diastolic blood-pressure and bodyweight. Maturitas 1:3, 1978

87.   National Center for Health Statistics: Blood pressure of adults by age and sex: United States 1960-1962. PHS Publication No. 1000, Series 11, No. 4. U.S. Government Printing Office, Washington, D.C., 1964

88.   McKay Hart D, Lindsay R, Purdie D: Vascular complications of long-term oestrogen therapy. Front Horm Res 5:174, 1978

89.   Weiss NS: Relationship of menopause to serum cholesterol and arterial blood pressure: The United States health examination survey of adults. Am J Epidemiol 96:237, 1972

90.   von Eiff AW: Bloodpressure and estrogens. Front Horm Res 3:177, 1975

91.   Fisch IR, Frank J: Oral contraceptives and blood pressure. JAMA 237:2499, 1977

92.   Stern PM, Brown BW, Haskell WL, et al.: Cardiovascular risk and use of estrogens or estrogen-progestagen combinations. JAMA 235:811, 1976

93.   Oral contraceptives and health: An interim report from the oral contraception study of the Royal College of General Practitioners. London, Pitman Medical, 1974

94.   Notelovitz M: Effect of natural oestrogens on bloodpressure and weight in postmenopausal women. S Afr Med J 49:2251, 1975

95.   Spellacy WN, Birk SA: The effect of I.U.D.s, oral contraceptives, estrogens and progestogens on blood pressure. Am J Obstet Gynecol 112:912, 1972

96.   Pallas KG, Holzwarth GJ, Stern MP, Lucas CP: The effect of conjugated estrogens on the renin-angiotensin system. J Clin Endocrinol Metab 44:1061, 1977

97.   Erkkola R, Lammintausta R, Punnonen R, Rauramo L: The effect of estriol succinate on plasma renin activity and urinary aldosterone in postmenopausal women. Maturitas 1:9, 1978

98.   Kreek MJ, Wisor E, Sleisenger MH, et al.: Idiopathic cholestasis of pregnancy: the response to challenge with the synthetic estrogen, ethinyl estradiol. N Engl J Med 277:1391, 1967

99.   Lynn J, Williams LF, O'Brien J, et al.: Efforts of estrogen upon bile; implications with respect to gallstone formation. Ann Surg 178:514, 1973

100.   Goldzieher JW, Chenault CG, de la Pena A, Dozier TS, Kraemer DC: Comparative studies of the ethynyl estrogens used in oral contraceptives. VI. Effects with and without progestational agents on carbohydrate metabolism in humans, baboons, and beagles. Fertil Steril 30:146, 1978

101.   Yen SSC, Vela P: Carbohydrate metabolism and long-term use of oral contraceptives. J Reprod Med 3:25, 1969

102.   Kalkhoff RK: Effects of oral contraceptive agents on carbohydrate metabolism. J Steroid Biochem 6:949, 1975

103.   Spellacy WN, Buhi WC, Birk SA: The effect of estrogens on carbohydrate metabolism: glucose, insulin, and growth hormone studies on one hundred and seventy one women ingesting premarin, mestranol, and ethinyl estradiol for six months. Am J Obstet Gynecol 114:378, 1972

104.   Beck P, Venable RL, Hoff DL: Mutual modification of glucose-stimulated serum insulin responses in female rhesus monkeys by ethinyl estradiol and nortestosterone derivatives. J Clin Endocrinol Metab 41:44, 1975

105.   Thom M, Chakravarti S, Oram DH, Studd JWW: Effect of hormone replacement therapy on glucose tolerance in postmenopausal women. Br J Obstet Gynaecol 84:776, 1976

106.   Notelovitz M: Metabolic effect of conjugated oestrogens on glucose tolerance. S Afr Med J 48:2599, 1974

107.   Notelovitz M: The effect of long-term oestrogen replacement therapy on glucose and lipid metabolism in postmenopausal women. S Afr Med J 50:2001, 1976

108.   Goldzieher JW, Villegas-Castrejon H, Cervantes A, Maqueo M, Siperstein M: Absence of diabetic capillary microangiopathy in oral contraceptive users with glucose intolerance. Obstet Gynecol 51:89, 1978

109.   Utian WH: Application of cost-effectiveness analysis to postmenopausal estrogen therapy. Front Horm Res 5:26, 1978

110.   Bush JW, Chen MM, Patrick DL: Health status index in cost-effectiveness analysis of PKU program. In Berg RL (ed): Health Status Indices. Chicago, Hospital Research and Educational Trust, 1973

111.   Weinstein MC, Stason WB: Foundations of cost-effectiveness analysis for health and medical practices. N Engl J Med 296:716, 1977

112.   Bunker JP, Barnes BA, Mosteller F: Costs, Risks and Benefits of Surgery. New York, Oxford University Press, 1977

113.   Aitken JM: Bone metabolism in post-menopausal women. In Beard R (ed): The Menopause. Lancaster, MTP Press, 1976, p. 95

114.   Dewhurst CJ: Financial implications of hormone replacement therapy. In Campbell S (ed): The Management of the Menopause and Postmenopausal Years. Lancaster, MTP Press, 1976, p. 429

9
Selective Pharmacotherapy After Menopause

The selection of pharmacologic agents, hormonal and nonhormonal, for use after menopause needs to be specific. Misuse or abuse of drugs can no longer be justified. This does not imply that physicians and patients should shun their use, an opposite extreme that also cannot be supported. Provided a definitive indication exists, and the basic principles of drug therapy are obeyed, including follow-up requirements, then the use of such agents will often generate extremely gratifying results and should not be unduly withheld.

The hormonal agents will be described specifically in relation to perimenopausal use. Nonhormonal drugs of value after menopause will be listed for the sake of completeness, although any major review is beyond the bounds of this monograph.

SEX HORMONES

The objective of this section is to provide information about the sex hormones that is clinically relevant. Following definition and classification, the question of indications, contraindications, selection of drugs, choice of route of administration, and dosage will be addressed.

Estrogens

DEFINITION   The estrogens are cyclopentanoperhydrophenanthrene derivatives similar to all steroid hormones, but are typified by having 18 carbon atoms, an aromatic A ring, and an associated phenolic hydroxyl group at carbon position 3. There are no estrogens known that do not contain an aromatic ring. Usually defined as substances responsible for producing estrus or heat and uterine enlargement in castrated animals, they are better characterized as the "hormones of femininity" capable of producing characteristic biologic effects on specific tissues such as vaginal epithelium, endometrium, and breast.[1,2]

PRACTICAL CLASSIFICATION   The estrogenic activity of a substance was believed to be related to the dose of substance administered and the specific response observed, but not to the actual type of estrogen given. There is an expanding literature, however, to suggest that different estrogens have different pharmacologic effects, even when equivalent doses of different estrogens are administered.[3-5] The selection of a drug for long-term therapy has thus become more difficult. This is an area still requiring considerable research.

The classification of estrogens in general use divides them into "natural" and "synthetic" types, an unfortunate situation, for natural estrogens may be synthesized and synthetic estrogens may be natural. The following generic classification, proposed for its greater clinical application, includes the most frequently listed estrogens.[6]

1. Conjugated steroidal estrogens
    Estrones: conjugated equine estrogens
                  esterified estrogens
                  piperazine estrone sulphate
    Estradiols: estradiol cypionate
                  estradiol valerate
                  micronized 17 β -estradiol
    Estriols: estriol
                  estriol hemisuccinate
2. Nonconjugated steroidal estrogens
                  17-Ethinyl-estradiol
                  17-Ethinyl-estradiol-3-methyl ether (mestranol)
                  17-Ethinyl-estradiol-3-cyclopentoether (quinestrol)
3. Estrogen analogues (nonsteroids)
                  benzestrol
                  cholorotrianisene
                  dienestrol
                  diethylstilbestrol
                  hexestrol
                  methallenestril
                  P1496[5]
                  promethestrol diproprorionate

Most of the above generic drugs are available under a number of trade names. The actual availability in different countries is, of course, dependent upon agencies such as the FDA in the United States and counterparts elsewhere. Moreover, not all these drugs are orally active, a subject to be discussed further below.

INDICATIONS   The following patients are those in whom estrogen may be indicated for the potential benefits previously described.[6]

1. Ovarian failure in the adult female, whether spontaneous or due to surgery, radiation, immunosuppressive disease, premature ovarian failure or pituitary failure.
2. Specific climacteric symptoms — hot flushes and vaginal atrophy.

3. Kraurosis vulvae (atrophy of vulva) and atrophic urethritis.

The sexually immature, prepubertal female with hypogonadism is also a candidate for estrogen replacement therapy. In this instance, the purpose of therapy is to assist the individual to achieve full sexual maturation and the closure of the epiphyses.

The advantages and disadvantages of long-term estrogen replacement therapy are evaluated in Chapter 8.

CONTRAINDICATIONS   Estrogens, under ordinary circumstances, should not be given to patients with the following:

1. Known or suspected breast or uterine cancer or any estrogen-dependent tumor.
2. Strong family history of estrogen-dependent neoplasia.
3. Abnormal genital bleeding that has not been diagnosed.
4. Previous or present thromboembolism or severe thrombophlebitis.
5. Dubin-Johnson syndrome (chronic idiopathic jaundice).
6. Acute liver disease.[7]

In addition, the presence of the following should lead to careful evaluation before estrogen prescription or proscription.

1. Uterine fibromyomata
2. Hyperlipidemia or hypercholesterolemia
3. Severe varicose veins
4. Chronic hepatic dysfunction
5. Diabetes mellitus
6. Porphyria
7. Severe hypertension

Finally, the combination of risk-factors such as obesity, varicosities, and heavy smoking could be additive and considered contraindications to estrogen therapy. These factors are also discussed in depth in Chapter 8.

CLINICAL USE

Drug Selection   It has already been emphasized that currently available information on estrogen risks influences the decision on which drug to use. At the present time, it would appear that a conjugated steroidal estrogen would be more appropriate for use in the postmenopausal female. Alternatively, it seems that the synthetic unconjugated steroids (ethinyl-estradiol and derivates) are associated with more side effects (see Chapter 8).[7] The following orally active substances have the best documentation for use.

Conjugated estrogens. These preparations contain not less than 50 percent and not more than 65 percent of sodium estrone sulfate, and not less than 20 percent and not more than 35 percent of sodium equilin sulfate, calculated on the basis of the total conjugated estrogens present. The conjugated equine estrogens are water-soluble estrogens derived from pregnant mares' urine, and are available as oral tablets of 0.3 mg, 0.625 mg, 1.25 mg, and 2.5 mg.

Esterified estrogens. These are similar to conjugated estrogens but contain 75 to 85 percent sodium estrone sulfate, and not more than 15 percent of sodium equilin sulfate, calculated on the same basis. They also contain less 17 α -estradiol, 17 α -dihydroequilin and 17 α -dihydroequilenin than do formulations of conjugated equine estrogens. They are available in 0.3 mg, 0.625 mg, 1.25 mg, and 2.5 mg tablets.

Piperazine estrone sulfate. This preparation is crystalline estrone solubilized as the sulfate and stabilized with piperazine. It is available usually in 0.625 mg, 1.25 mg, 2.5 mg, and 5.0 mg tablets.

Estradiol valerate. This is a fatty acid ester of the naturally occurring estradiol. The valeric acid ester is excreted via the lungs. Estradiol valerate is available in 1 mg and 2 mg tablets.

Estriol hemisuccinate. This is the hemisuccinate ester of naturally occurring estriol and is available in 1 mg and 2 mg tablets.

Estradiol. Estradiol is the most potent natural estrogen. 17 β -estradiol that has been micronized has been demonstrated to be rapidly and effectively absorbed from the gastrointestinal tract.[8] It is available in 1 mg and 2 mg tablets.

Estriol. This is available in its natural form in 1 mg and 2 mg tablets. It is becoming popular because of its weak endometrial proliferation effect.[9]

Route of Administration   The alternatives to oral estrogens are aqueous or oily solutions for intramuscular injection, pellets for subcutaneous implantation, or creams for skin or vaginal application. Two forms of vaginal estrogen cream are available, one with conjugated estrogens and the other with dienestrol.

Orally administered estrogens are preferable to implants or injections for the following reasons:

1.   Treatment can be rapidly stopped for any reason.
2.   The dose can be more precisely controlled.
3.   Therapy can be cyclic, and progestogen can be added.
4.   Swallowing a tablet is painless.
5.   Medication is cheaper and can be self-administered.[6,10]

Certain other factors may influence the mode of administration, including recent information which shows that vaginal creams[11] or topical skin creams[12] are associated with absorption rates equivalent to the oral route. Moreover, avoidance of the gastrointestinal tract also eliminates the first liver passage of the drug and this may influence plasma and tissue levels and hence the metabolic properties of the drug. For example, the primary effect of orally administered micronized 17 β-estradiol is an elevation of serum estrone with a much less significant increase in estradiol.[8] This is probably due to the conversion of estradiol to estrone in the small bowel. Micronized 17 β-estradiol given by the vaginal route, however, does not undergo conversion and estradiol is the primary serum estrogen seen.[11] Similar differences have been demonstrated for estriol. When administered vaginally it appears to be conjugated less rapidly, thus rendering it more biologically potent.[13] Further research in this area is in progress, and the results could well influence practical management in the future.[14]

Although the author is not personally in favor of hormonal implants, the above findings do support their recognized use.[15] Implants can be inserted into the subcutaneous fat of the anterior abdominal wall (about two inches above the inguinal ligament) or into the upper, outer quadrant of the buttock. Strict asepsis is mandatory. Skin is cleansed with an acceptable operative skin preparation and a small area appropriately draped. Anesthesia is induced by local injection.

The preferred technique is to utilize a trochar and cannula, the full length of which is forced through the anesthetized skin into the subcutaneous tissues. The implant should be handled with sterile instruments only. The trochar is removed, the pellet inserted into the cannula, and then the trochar replaced to plunge the implant to the full length of the cannula. Following withdrawal of trochar and cannula, a waterproof sterile dressing is placed on the wound and the patient advised to keep the area dry for 48 hours.

Dosage   The actual selection of dose should be individualized according to the specific indication and the therapeutic response. In usual clinical practice, for example, if short-term relief of symptoms is required, an empirical low dose is prescribed, and increased if symptoms fail to respond.

Normally, the lowest possible dose should be administered to obtain the desired relief. According to FDA recommendations, this should be administered for the shortest possible time. But how does one estimate the lowest effective dose? A measure commonly used to compare estrogens is the "proliferative dose." This is the total dose that will produce full endometrial proliferation in a previously unstimulated or gonadectomized animal. The following are the proliferative doses of some commonly used oral estrogens.

Name	Proliferative dose in mg
Chlorotrianisene	over 100
Conjugated equine estrogens	60-80
Diethylstilbestrol	20-30
Ethinyl-estradiol	2
Estradiol valerate	60
Estriol	120-150
Mestranol	2
Quinestrol	2

Dosage may need to be changed for long-term therapy aimed at specific metabolic parameters. The following factors should be borne in mind as possible aids to dosage selection:

Symptom Response.   The only specific symptom of estrogen deficiency is the hot flush. The patient should keep a "flush count" every day and note the response to treatment. Conjugated equine estrogen 0.625 mg, micronized 17 β-estradiol 1 mg, estradiol valerate 1 mg, estriol 2 mg, or estriol succinate 4 mg are usually sufficient to relieve hot flushes in most patients when given in a daily dose.[7,9,16-20]

Change in Hormonal Cytology.   There is nothing to be gained by increasing doses of exogenous estrogen in an attempt to increase the vaginal cornification index or superficial cell count. The concept of a "femininity index" on the vaginal smear is an erroneous one that has already been perpetuated for too long; the vaginal smear is treated and not the patient! All that is required is a dose of estrogen sufficient to remove the parabasal cells.[21] The reason for this was discussed in Chapter 4.

FSH and LH Response.   Contrary to expectations, exogenous estrogen treatment will not always reduce pituitary gonadotropin (FSH and LH) values to premenopausal levels.[8,22] It is not possible, therefore, to calculate a therapeutic dose of estrogen by looking at the gonadotropin response.

Response of Fasting Plasma and Urinary Calcium Levels.   It is possible that the potency of estrogenic preparations and the potential bone effect can be predicted by the response of the fasting plasma or urinary calcium to estrogen therapy.[23] Ovarian removal results in negative calcium balance; estrogen therapy produces a positive calcium balance.[3,23]

Cyclicity   It is now generally accepted that therapy should be cyclic, even in a patient without a uterus. This would allow the estrogenic-induced tissue buildup a chance to reduce in amount (e.g., endometrium, breast), and is more physiologic than a constant tonic estrogen level. A convenient regime is to prescribe tablets from the first to the twenty-fifth of each month, leaving the latter part of the month pill-free.[10]

Progestin therapy is frequently recommended, although evidence for the value of such therapy is not yet available. It is possible that progestin will block estrogen receptors and limit over-growth of tissue.[24] Progestin, when prescribed, should be given with the last seven to ten days of estrogen therapy. At this point in time, selection of drug and dose has to be based on empirical standards.

RISKS AND SIDE EFFECTS   The possible risk of estrogen usage and the side effects have been fully described in Chapter 8.

Progestogens

DEFINITION   Progesterone is a C-21 steroid hormone of the pregnane series. It is the hormone of pregnancy. Biologically it is remarkably inert unless tissues have been previously primed with estrogens.[1] Synthetic compounds with progesterone-like effects are called progestogens (progestins).

CLASSIFICATION AND DESCRIPTION   Progesterone and the dihydroprogesterones are the only known naturally occurring progestational agents.[1] These are relatively inactive when taken by mouth. Modification of the progesterone molecule has proved the basis for some synthetic progestogens. Moreover, testosterone, appropriately modified, has progestational activity. Thus 19 nortestosterone (19 norethisterone) forms a root compound for many of the oral progestogens.

It is most important to remember the derivation of the progestogens because these synthetic compounds do not all have a spectrum of activity identical to progesterone. In particular, those compounds derived from testosterone can induce androgenic effects.

The following are the most well-known of the orally active progestational compounds:[2]

1. Progesterone derivatives
   dydrogesterone (6-dehydroretroprogesterone)
2. Acetoxyprogesterone derivatives
   medroxyprogesterone acetate
   megestrol acetate
3. 19 nortestosterone derivatives and relatives
   chlormadinone acetate
   ethynodiol diacetate
   lynestrenol (3-desoxonorethindrone)
   norethindrone (norethisterone)
   norethindrone acetate
   norethynodrel
   norgestrel
   norgestrienone

Many of the above compounds are only available in combination with estrogens as the oral contraceptive. Others may or may not be available in specific countries depending on local regulations. They have been well reviewed by Edgren.[2] The following oral progestogens, in the experience of the author, are the most frequently used after menopause:

Medroxyprogesterone acetate. Available in 2.5- and 10-mg tablets, this compound is extremely popular because of its low androgenic potential. It is 6 α-methyl-17 α-acetoxy progesterone.

Megestrol acetate. Available in 20-mg tablets, this is the $\triangle$ 6 derivative of medroxyprogesterone and also has low androgenicity.

Dydrogesterone. Available in 5- and 10-mg tablets, it is of low androgenic potential.

Norethindrone. Available in 5-mg tablets, it is more likely to induce androgenic effects because it is the 17 α-ethinyl derivative of 19-nortestosterone.

CLINICAL USE AND INDICATIONS
Indications   The indications and contraindications for progestogens after menopause are still under review. Despite considerable research in progress, little solid data is yet available. Practically speaking, the most specific indication for progestogens after menopause is in cyclic combination with estrogen, for the following reasons.

Rationale   During the follicular phase of a normal menstrual cycle the estrogen-responsive endometrium proliferates and increases in thickness by as much as tenfold. After ovulation the total endometrial height is relatively fixed, although estrogen continues to be available. This inhibition of further growth is considered to be related to the presence of increasing amounts of progesterone. The relationship between estrogen, endometrial hyperplasia, uterine cancer, and the possible role for progestogens is discussed in depth in Chapter 8.

The endometrial response to the progestogens is variable, depending upon the preexisting estrogenic buildup, and the type of progestogen administered. In general, progestogen therapy is associated with a divergence between glandular and stromal development. The glands become atrophic and the stroma proliferates, demonstrating a pseudo-decidual change.[2] It is this particular property which makes the progestogens so valuable as an adjunct to estrogen therapy after menopause.

Clinical experience has tended to bear out expectations. Progestogens have been reported to convert hyperplastic endometrium to the normal state,[25] on a basis of mitotic arrest with decrease in RNA and

DNA synthesis similar to that which occurs in the normal cyclic regressive endometrium.[26] There are several reports of the clinical response of this alteration in endometrium, notably a lower incidence of abnormal bleeding,[27] with a significant reduction in the incidence of endometrial hyperplasia.[28-30] Although no definitive evidence exists for a reduction in the postmenopausal estrogen-induced increase in endometrial cancer by use of progestogens, Gambrell has suggested that the possibility may exist.[30,31]

DRUG SELECTION AND DOSE   The progestogens listed above are all orally active, the preferred route after menopause. There is little evidence to favor one drug type over another except for the androgenic aspect described.

Progestogens, when used with estrogens, are normally prescribed for the final 7 to 10 days of a 21- to 25-day estrogen course. The dosage depends upon the drug selected; for example, the usual dose of medroxyprogesterone acetate is 10 mg per day and for norethindrone acetate it is 5 mg.

CONTRAINDICATIONS AND RISKS   There are no known absolute contraindications for progestogens after the menopause (see Chapter 8), but the following should be considered as possible relative contraindications:

1.   Previous or present thromboembolism or severe thrombophlebitis
2.   Liver dysfunction or disease
3.   Undiagnosed uterine bleeding

COMBINATIONS OF ESTROGEN WITH PROGESTOGEN
Estrogen-progestogen combinations, as in oral contraceptive formulations, are not generally favored or advised after menopause. These combination pills are too restrictive in terms of drug type and dose and it is more preferable to select and administer estrogens and progestogens on an individual basis.

Androgens

Since the introduction of the orally-active progestational agents, the androgens have, in the opinion of the author, lost their indication for use in the treatment of climacteric-related problems. For this reason, these drugs will not be dealt with further. The advantage of the androgens was the ability to induce a feeling of well-being and improve libido; the cost to the patient was often hirsutism, acne, and other signs of virilism.

NONHORMONAL DRUGS

Nonhormonal drugs have a secondary role in the management of the climacteric syndrome. That is, specific hormone-dependent symptoms or metabolic factors respond best to selected hormones and should be treated primarily with these substances provided no contraindication to their use exists. Symptoms that develop as a result of psycho-socio-cultural factors necessitate an educational and psychotherapeutic approach, with the use of drugs as an adjunct only. It is of course obvious that unexplained symptoms should always be investigated for a specific cause, and be treated according to accepted principles of practice dependent upon that cause.

There are specific instances when nonhormonal drugs may be indicated in the management of the climacteric syndrome and these situations include:

1. The patient in whom sex-steroid therapy is contraindicated.
2. The patient who does not respond to sex-steroid therapy.
3. The patient who does not want hormone therapy but does request symptom relief.
4. The patient who cannot tolerate sex steroids because of side effects such as nausea or fluid retention.

The selection of a nonhormonal drug for treatment of the climacteric syndrome is based more on empirical observation than on satisfactory documentation for therapeutic effect. The literature is striking for its paucity of well-controlled, randomized, double-blind, prospective studies of the therapeutic efficacy of nonhormonal agents. A brief discussion follows on some of the more frequently prescribed drugs or groups of drugs.

Sedatives

Sedatives may help in reducing the number of hot flushes. They are less useful for the symptoms associated with irritability and emotional upset. Clinical experience appears to have been greater with the barbiturate sedatives than with the nonbarbiturates. In particular, phenobarbital USP, alone or in combination with other drugs, seems to be effective. For example, based on the concept that functional disorders may involve hyperactivity of the sympathetic and parasympathetic nervous systems, phenobarbital USP 20 to 40 mg is combined with ergotamine tartrate, a sympathetic inhibitor, and levorotatory alkaloids of belladonna, a parasympathetic inhibitor. In the author's personal experience, this combination is less effective than estrogen in relief of hot flushes, but is a satisfactory alternate when estrogens cannot be used. It is commercially available as Bellergal tablets.

Tranquilizers

The tranquilizers now comprise a large group of drugs, the description of which is outside the scope of this monograph. It can be stated that these drugs have often been abused in relation to the postmenopausal patient, with excessive use, and all too often in the absence of a well-defined indication. Nonetheless, in appropriately selected patients tranquilizers are of value as adjuncts to educational and psychotherapeutic programs, particularly in the presence of excessive anxiety, irritability, insomnia, and related agitational states.

The most frequently prescribed drugs include diazepam (Valium), chlordiazepoxide (Librium), benezodiazepine (Ativan), hydroxyzine (Atarax), meprobamate, and some of the phenothiazines. The reader is advised to refer to standard texts for current prescribing practices relating to these drugs.

Antidepressants

Similar remarks apply to the antidepressants as for the tranquilizers discussed above. These drugs are indicated for true psychiatric depression. They are less likely to be of value in situations with marginal mood changes not severe enough to be classified as depression. Among the most commonly used antidepressants are amitriptyline (Elavil), some of the phenothiazines, monoamine oxidase inhibitors (e.g., phenelzine sulfate — Nardil; tranylcypromine sulfate — Parnate), the dibenzoxepin tricyclic compounds (doxepin HCL — Sinequan), and the imipramines (imipramine pamoate — Tofranil).

Clonidine

Clonidine, an imidazoline derivative, is worthy of discussion because of the attention it has received as an alternate to estrogen in the treatment of hot flushes. Introduced in low dose as an antimigraine drug,[32] and in higher dose as an antihypertensive,[33,34] clonidine was reported by Clayden to be effective in reducing perimenopausal flushing.[35,36] Clonidine appears to inhibit sympathetic nervous system function at least in part by interaction with a central alpha adrenergic receptor.[37]

Personal experience has been less promising, and a recent double-blind crossover trial of clonidine failed to show any effect of the drug on menopausal flushing.[38] Nonetheless, further research is indicated both to elucidate the cause of the hot flush and to find suitable nonhormonal forms of medication.

Propranolol

Propranolol, a drug which causes both central and peripheral beta-blockade, has also been studied for its effect on menopausal hot flushes, but was shown to be no more effective than a placebo.[39]

Vitamin B-6 (Pyridoxine)

As in the oral contraceptive, there is some evidence to show that ethinyl-estradiol and possibly progestogens lead to a disturbance of tryptophan metabolism and a deficiency of vitamin B-6 (pyridoxine).[40,41,42] Adams el al. have reported that the clinical consequences include depression, emotional instability, fatigue, disturbances in concentration, and loss of libido.[41] The same problem has been reported by Haspels et al. to occur in postmenopausal women on estrogen therapy.[43] These symptoms apparently respond to vitamin B-6, 250 mg per day.[41,43] Altered tryptophan metabolism with sex-steroid therapy appears to warrant further investigation.

References

1.   Henzl MR: Natural and synethic female sex hormones. In Yen SSC, Jaffe RB (eds): Reproductive Endocrinology. Philadelphia, Saunders, 1978

2.   Edgren RA: Comparative effects of new progestogens. In Gold JJ (ed): Gynecologic Endocrinology. Maryland, Harper and Row, 1975

3.   Utian WH: Effects of oophorectomy and subsequent oestrogen therapy on plasma calcium and phosphorus. S Afr J Gynaecol Obstet 10:8, 1972

4.   Utian WH: Effects of oophorectomy and oestrogen therapy on serum cholesterol. Int J Gynaecol Obstet 10:95, 1972

5.   Utian WH: Comparative trial of P1496, a new non-steroidal oestrogen-analogue. Br Med J 1:579, 1973

6.   Utian WH: Estrogen replacement in the menopause. In Wynn R (ed): Obstetrics and Gynecology Annual. New York, Appleton, 1979

7.   Lauritzen C: The management of the premenopausal and the postmenopausal patient. Front Horm Res 2:2, 1973

8.   Yen SSC, Martin PL, Burnier AM, et al.: Circulatiñg estradiol, estrone and gonadotropin levels following the administration of orally active 17 β -estradiol in postmenopausal women. J Clin Endocrinol Metab 40:518, 1975

9.   Tzingounis VA, Aksu MF, Greenblatt RB: Estriol in the management of the menopause. JAMA 239:1638, 1978

10.   Utian WH: The scientific basis for postmenopausal estrogen therapy: the management of specific symptoms and rationale for long-term replacement. In Beard R (ed): The Menopause. Lancaster, MTP Press, 1976, p. 1975

11.   Rigg LA, Hermann H, Yen SSC: Absorption of estrogens from vaginal creams. N Engl J Med 298:195, 1978

12.   Loeper J, Loeper J, Ohlghiesser C, et al.: The influence of estrogen therapy on triglycerides. Importance of the choice of substance and the route of administration. Nouv Presse Med 6:2747, 1977

13.   Schiff I, Wentworth B, Koos B, Ryan KJ, Tulchinsky D: Effect of estriol administration on the hypogonadal woman. Fertil Steril 30:278, 1978

14.   Sitruk-Ware R: Personal communication. Percutaneous absorption of estrogenic steroids, 1978

15.   Studd JWW: Hormone implants in the climacteric syndrome. In Campbell S (ed): The Management of the Menopause. Lancaster, MTP Press, 1976, p 383

16.   Lozman H, Barlow AL, Levitt DG: Piperazine estrone sulfate and conjugated estrogens equine in the treatment of the menopausal syndrome. South Med J 64:1143, 1971

17.   Campbell S, Whitehead M: In Greenblatt RB, Studd JWW (eds): Clinics in Obstetrics and Gynecology, Vol 4, No. 1. Philadelphia, Saunders, 1977

18.   Kullander S, Svanberg L: On climacteric symptoms and their treatment with a new non-steroidal estrogen. Int J Gynaecol Obstet 13:277, 1975

19.   Velikay L: The oral treatment of the climacteric syndrome with oestradiol valerate. Wien Klin Wochenschr 80:229, 1968

20.   Dapunt O: The treatment of climacteric symptoms with oestradiol valerate. Med Klin 62:1356, 1967

21.   Utian WH: Use of vaginal smear in assessment of oestrogenic status of oophorectomized females. S Afr Med J 44:69, 1970

22.   Utian WH, Katz M, Davey DA, Carr PJ: Effect of premenopausal castration and incremental dosages of conjugated equine estrogens on plasma follicle stimulating hormone, luteinizing hormone, and estradiol. Am J Obstet Gynecol 132:297, 1978

23.   Utian WH; Osteoporosis, oestrogens and oophorectomy; proposed new test of oestrogenic potency. S Afr Med J 49:433, 1975

24.   Hsueh AJW, Peck EJ, Clark JH: Control of uterine estrogen receptor levels by progesterone. Endocrinology 98:438, 1976

25.   Wentz WB: Progestin therapy for endometrial hyperplasia. Gynecol Oncol 2:362, 1974

26.   Richart RM, Ferenczy A: Endometrial morphologic response to hormonal environment. Gynecol Oncol 2:180, 1974

27.   Martin PL, Burnier AM, Segre EJ, Huix FJ: Graded sequential therapy in the menopause: a double-blind study. Am J Obstet Gynecol 111:178, 1971

28.   Benjamin I, Block RE: Endometrial response to estrogen and progesterone therapy in patients with gonadal dysgenesis. Obstet Gynecol 50:136, 1977

29.   Stryker JC: Use of hormones in women over forty. Clin Obstet Gynecol 20:155, 1977

30.   Gambrell RD: Estrogens, progestogens and endometrial cancer. In van Keep PA, Greenblatt RB, Albeaux-Fernet M (eds): Consensus on Menopause Research. Lancaster, MTP Press, 1976, p. 152

31.   Gambrell RD: The prevention of endometrial cancer in postmenopausal women with progestogens. Maturitas 1:107, 1978

32.   Shafar J, Tallett ER, Knowlson PA: Evaluation of clonidine in prophylaxis of migraine. Double-blind trial and follow-up. Lancet 1:403, 1972

33.   Haeusler G: Cardiovascular regulation by central adrenergic mechanisms and its alteration by hypotensive drugs. Circ Res Suppl 36-37:223, 1975

34.   van Zwieten PA: The central action of antihypertensive drugs mediated by central α -receptors. J Pharm Pharmacol 25:89, 1973

35.   Clayden JR: Effect of clonidine on menopausal flushing. Lancet 2:1361, 1972

36.   Clayden JR, Bell JW, Pollard P: Menopausal flushing — double-blind trial of a non-hormonal medication. Br Med J 1:409, 1974

37.   Metz SA, Halter JB, Porte D, Robertson RP: Suppression of plasma catecholamines and flushing by clonidine in man. J Clin Endocrinol Metab 46:83, 1978

38.   Lindsay R, Hart DM: Failure of response of menopausal vasomotor symptoms to clonidine. Maturitas 1:21, 1978

39.   Coope J, Williams S, Patterson JS: A study of the effectiveness of propranolol in menopausal hot flushes. Br J Obstet Gynaecol 85:472, 1978

40.   Rose DP: Excretion of xanthurenic acid in the urine of women taking progestogen-oestrogen preparations. Nature 210:196, 1966

41.   Adams PW, Rose DP, Folkard J, et al.: Effect of vitamin B_6 upon depression associated with oral contraception. Lancet 1:897, 1973

42.   Coelingh Bennink HJT, Schreurs WHP: Disturbance of tryptophan metabolism and its correction during hormonal contraception. Contraception 9:347, 1974

43.   Haspels AA, Coelingh Bennink HJT, Schreurs WHP: Disturbance of tryptophan metabolism and its correction during oestrogen treatment in postmenopausal women. Maturitas 1:15, 1978

10
Practical Aspects of Clinical Care

Areas of clinical significance have been alluded to in the preceding text. The present objective is to consolidate this information into practical guidelines for clinical care, and to consider some special problems that arise in the management of the woman after menopause. Observation of the general principles outlined should not only enhance and improve clinical results, but, of equal importance, provide support for the physician in the handling of a provocative and emotive area of patient care.

DIAGNOSIS OF CLIMACTERIC
Diagnosing Climacteric Before Menopause

It is often difficult to confirm that a patient has entered climacteric if she has not yet become menopausal. Symptoms that should promote a high index of suspicion include:

1. Alterations in menstrual pattern—specifically, irregular frequency of periods, decreased menstrual flow, or evidence of anovulation which may then be associated with hypermenorrhea.
2. The onset of hot flushes.

Unfortunately, there are no satisfactory practical laboratory tests of confirmatory value. Plasma gonadotropins may be marginally elevated, but not sufficiently to be of clinical use. Similarly, dynamic tests of hormonal function are of no diagnostic help.

Confirming Menopause

An interval of six months or more of secondary amenorrhea in a woman over the age of 50 is usually diagnostic of menopause, especially if this is accompanied by the development of hot flushes and/or a low estrogen profile on physical examination (e.g., atrophic vaginal smear, absence of cervical mucus, atrophic endometrium on biopsy). In younger women the menses should be absent for at least one year to diagnose menopause with the same degree of confidence.

A negative response to a progestogen challenge test (for example, medroxyprogesterone acetate 10 mg tablets orally for 7 days) is confirmatory of low estrogen production and in most instances is the only special test necessary. If some doubt exists, and urgent diagnostic confirmation is requested, the measurement of the plasma FSH level is an adequate adjunct.

Differential Diagnosis of Amenorrhea

Diagnostic difficulty often arises when a younger woman, say in her thirties or early forties, presents with secondary amenorrhea. Indeed, this is one of the most frequent symptoms for referral to a gynecologic endocrine unit.[1] There are many possible causes for primary[2,3] and secondary amenorrhea[4,5] and these have been the subject of excellent reviews.[6,7]

Jacobs and co-investigators present an extremely practical approach to the diagnosis of secondary amenorrhea based on a series of steps designed to evaluate pathology, but in each instance directed toward treatment.[1] The therapy-oriented protocol for diagnosis of secondary amenorrhea in Figure 10-1, modified from Jacobs et al., is the one used by the author and is self-explanatory. The paper by Jacobs et al. deserves reading.[1]

Diagnosing Menopause in Women on Oral Contraceptives

A special problem arises in the older woman on oral contraceptives who asks if she can discontinue the pill without fear of pregnancy. A diagnosis can be made if the pill is discontinued and then estrogen and FSH values are examined four weeks later.[8] It is pertinent to remember that only a postmenopausal FSH elevation can distinguish between an ovulatory LH surge and the menopause.

Diagnosis After Hysterectomy

The onset of hot flushes is the most frequent signal of ovarian failure after hysterectomy with conserved ovaries. The diagnosis is confirmed by measurement of the plasma FSH level.

MINIMAL REQUIREMENTS FOR INITIAL PREHORMONE THERAPY WORKUP

The administration of estrogen to a patient with a known contraindication, especially if this results in complications, could result in litigation. For this reason many physicians choose not to consider hor-

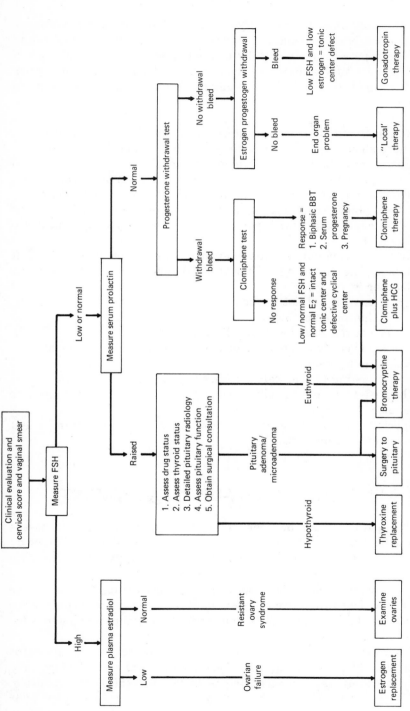

Figure 10-1. Protocol for cost-effective treatment-oriented diagnosis of secondary amenorrhea (Modified from Jacobs et al.: Horm Res 6:268, 1975).

mone therapy. This attitude is too defensive, however, and the observation of a few basic precautions suffices to eliminate unjustifiable suits.

Every patient must be fully evaluated as to the general state of health by currently accepted methods including full history and physical examination (Table 10-1). In particular, the following points are of importance:

1. An indication for treatment must exist (see Chapters 8 and 9).
2. There should be no contraindications to estrogen (Chapter 9).
3. Menopause should be confirmed, preferably by a minimum of six months' amenorrhea and the presence of specific estrogen deficiency symptoms, or elevated plasma FSH and low estrogens.
4. A full general examination including blood pressure, breast and pelvic examination with cervical and vaginal cytologic smears is essential.
5. An attempt should be made to evaluate the degree of estrogen deficiency. The following adjuncts to diagnosis were discussed in Chapter 9:
    a. severity of hot flushes
    b. hormonal cytology
    c. plasma FSH level (usually necessary)
    d. urinary estrogen and/or plasma estradiol levels (usually unnecessary)
    e. fasting plasma calcium (rarely indicated)
6. The patient should be fully informed (see below) and must agree to regular checkups.
7. Special and more frequent attention must be given to the patient considered to be at risk.[9]

MINIMAL FOLLOW-UP REQUIREMENTS

The patient must be seen at least every six months to assess general health, clinical response, and adequacy of dosage. Follow-up visits should include, minimally, breast and pelvic examinations with cytology, and blood pressure checkup (Table 10-2).

An annual endometrial biopsy is a wise precaution in view of the cancer risk. This procedure in itself, however, needs to be examined for its cost: benefit value as well as to its indications if a progestogen is being used.

There are various methods for obtaining endometrial specimens for cytologic or histologic diagnosis of the endometrial state.[10] Most have not been widely used as screening tests because they are expensive, complicated, or unreliable. The best methods are as follows (page 166):

Table 10-1.   List of Important Factors in the Initial Workup Before prescribing Long-Term Hormone Therapy

History	Presenting symptoms or complaints
Family history	Heart disease
	Cancer of the breast, uterus or cervix
	Diabetes
Personal history	Menopausal age/menstrual pattern
	Vaginal Bleeding (esp. undiagnosed bleeding)
	Particulars of pregnancies
	Gynecological operations
	Breasts
	Heart disease
	Thromboembolic disorders
	Liver disease
	Diabetes
	Allergy and contraindications to drugs
	Family relationships and personal problems
Current disorders	Menopausal
	Hot flushes
	Bouts of perspiration
	Backache
	Psycho-socio-cultural
	Nervousness, irritability, headache, insomnia, depression, etc.
	Other factors
	Stress incontinence or prolapse
	Vaginal irritation
	Aches in bone or joints
	Sexual relations
	Frequency
	Satisfaction
	Pain
	Change in interest or desire
General physical examination—Note especially	Blood pressure
	Height and weight
	Breasts (mammography if necessary)
	Condition of skin, scalp hair, face.
Pelvic examination	
Laboratory examination	Urinalysis—sugar and protein
	Hematocrit/hemoglobin
	Cervical smear
	Hormone index on vaginal smear

Based on Groote Schuur Hospital Menopause Clinic Protocol, and on van Keep, Haspels: Oestrogen Therapy. Amsterdam, Excerpta Medica, 1977. Courtesy of Excerpta Medica.

Table 10-2. Recommended Biannual Follow-Up Procedures for Women on Long-Term Hormone Therapy.

History	Specifically any adverse effects
Physical	Especially:
	Blood pressure
	Height and weight
	Breast palpation
	Pelvic examination
Laboratory tests	Cervical and vaginal smear[*]
	Fasting and 2-hour glucose[*]
	Hemoglobin/hematocrit[†]
	Fasting plasma cholesterol and lipid analysis[*]
	Urinalysis
	Endometrial biopsy[*]
	Mammography[†]

[*]These procedures should be repeated once a year.
[†]Only to be undertaken when indicated.

Dilatation and Curretage   This remains the most effective method for obtaining endometrial tissue for cytologic and histologic evaluation and has an overall accuracy of 95 percent or better.[10] Unfortunately, this is not a practical screen for endometrial cancer and other methods have had to be developed.

Endometrial Biopsy   The so-called micro-curettage, effectively performed with a number of specifically designed instruments, for example, the Meigs or the Duncan endometrial biopsy curettes, suffers from one drawback: only a limited amount of tissue can be obtained, which makes the detection of localized lesions less reliable.[10]

Aspiration Biopsy   Vacuum aspiration of endometrial tissue (Vabra aspirator) was first described in 1968 by Jensen and Jensen.[11] Buchman et al. confirmed the value of the Vabra aspirator and the Novak suction curette in obtaining adequate endometrial specimens for histologic diagnosis from asymptomatic patients receiving estrogen.[12] The method is inadequate when endometrial atrophy is present;[10] otherwise a positive diagnosis can be made in up to 97 percent of cases with the Vabra aspirator.[13] Hutton et al. found the Isaacs cell sampler to be safe, quick, comfortable, and reliable.[14] Satisfactory aspirates for cytologic diagnosis were possible in 91 percent of patients and endometrial samples for histologic diagnosis in 79 percent. The author's personal preference is for the Vabra aspirator.

Irrigation Biopsy   Vooijs, based on a comprehensive survey of the literature, reported that this method is not a sufficiently reliable screening procedure because malignancy cannot be excluded even in the presence of a negative sample.[10]

Aspiration Cytology   The best alternative to endometrial aspiration would appear to be a direct aspiration of a sample for cytology from the cervical canal. The overall accuracy in the detection of endometrial cancer and its precursors is about 75 percent in experienced hands.[15]

PRESCRIBING DRUGS

Description of hormonal and nonhormonal drugs for perimenopausal use is dealt with in depth in Chapter 9.

Duration of Therapy

The duration of therapy is dependent upon variables previously enumerated and discussed. The patient is influenced by numerous factors such as attitudes of the doctor, discussions through the news media, experience of friends, and response to therapy. The recommendation of the doctor will of course depend upon his evaluation of the advantages and disadvantages of such therapy, and perhaps the degree of pressure exerted on him by the patient herself.[16]

Treating Adverse Effects

The incidence of estrogen-induced side effects is usually low, provided the drugs are correctly selected and prescribed. The type and severity of adverse effects will be influenced by individual patient idiosyncrasy, general health, selection of drug and dose, the mode of administration, and so on.

Major adverse effects of estrogens have been discussed in Chapter 8, and must be treated according to accepted medical principles. Minor side effects are not usually of serious consequence but do have considerable nuisance value. The following two symptoms are fairly frequent with estrogen therapy:

1.   Nausea occurs in up to 20 percent of patients during the first two to three months of therapy. Treatment may require reduction in estrogen dose but is usually successfully achieved by reassurance, advice

to take tablets with the evening meal, and prescription of antiemetic preparations.
2. Retention of excessive amounts of fluid may manifest as breast tenderness and/or weight gain. Reassurance, once again, is usually of value. Occasionally the dosage of estrogen will need reduction, or a change of preparation may be required. The use of diuretics is not recommended.

ADJUNCTS TO DRUG THERAPY

It is often gratifying to note the extent to which additional counseling can further enhance the quality of life of women seeking perimenopausal medical advice. The following are but a few areas in which judicious counseling can be of value:

1. Correct diet, particularly use of weight-reducing diets where indicated.
2. Total body care, including advice about oral and dental hygiene, cosmetics, and care of skin and nails.
3. Physical fitness programs. Selective exercise programs, both home plans and health studio plans, can be recommended following a satisfactory physical evaluation.
4. Marital counseling.
5. Psychosexual counseling.

INFORMING THE PATIENT

Under ideal circumstances, the patient contemplating hormone therapy after menopause should be able to evaluate the risks and benefits on a fully informed basis and then make her own decision whether to begin treatment or not. In practical terms this is almost impossible. No physician has the time, nor every patient the ability, to discuss the subject to the necessary extent on a one-to-one basis.

The Food and Drug Administration in the United States has attempted to circumvent this problem by requiring that a leaflet outlining the risks of sex steroids be given to each patient with every prescription of estrogen or progestogen.[17] In practice this often leads to rejection of therapy on a basis of misinterpretation of data.

There are in fact no easy answers to the process of informing the patient. The author has prepared a short book for the general population describing in lay language the information presented in this monograph.[18] Experience with such a manual has been extremely gratifying in that patients can be referred to detailed but simple explanations that can be read at leisure. Not only is time saved in office consultations, but the actual utilization of consultation time is enhanced by improved doctor-patient communication. Moreover, the woman's attention can be drawn to more personal components such as total body care, diet, and exercise without embarrassment to either physician or patient.

ROLE OF THE MENOPAUSE CLINIC

The value of a menopause clinic for centralization and control of estrogen therapy has been described by Utian.[16,19] In summary, the benefits are as follows:

1. The menopause clinic serves as a well-woman's clinic for middle-aged and older females. As a natural progression from family planning and prenatal programs, an opportunity is created to provide medical checkups for women of older age groups who may not otherwise be offered such services.
2. Screening programs for breast cancer, diabetes, hypertension, etc., can be introduced and coordinated for large populations.
3. Menopause experience is gathered in one center.
4. All medical and paramedical specialties (e.g., psychiatry, internal medicine, sociology, dietetics, etc.) can be coordinated and involved.
5. Estrogen therapy can be better controlled and evaluated on a short- or long-term basis.
6. Centralization of care can be made extremely cost-effective.
7. A menopause service can offer broad educational programs with a potential for better informing the patient and contributing to changed societal attitudes as well.
8. Research is a major component of a menopause clinic, and provides the best way to planning, developing, and coordinating prospective long-term evaluations of the effects of various hormone treatments. Indeed, this was the author's initial objective in establishing the Groote Schuur Hospital Menopause Clinic in 1967, probably the first example of its kind, and which has to date been highly successful in stimulating interdisciplinary long-term collaborative research.

INFLUENCE OF GOVERNMENTAL LEGISLATION ON PHYSICIANS' ATTITUDES AND THE DOCTOR–PATIENT RELATIONSHIP

The advent of the "estrogen debate" resulted in governmental agencies such as the FDA in the United States becoming directly involved. This led to a statement by the FDA that it "believes that the new findings linking postmenopausal estrogen administration to endometrial cancer must be considered carefully by every physician who prescribes these drugs and every patient who takes them."[17] Furthermore, the FDA insisted that a descriptive leaflet be inserted in the drug package for the patient so that she could be fully informed and able to participate in the decision whether or not to use estrogens.

There is a distinct danger that direct governmental agency intervention could interfere with the doctor-patient relationship. In particular, too little emphasis has been placed on the ability of the physician to balance the risk:benefit ratio for a specific patient and to make proper recommendations. Moreover, the limitation of the physician's discretion hampers his dialogue with the patient, and also raises the specter of mistrust and potential litigation on otherwise spurious grounds. Not surprisingly the stance of the FDA has been challenged and the outcome of this debate, yet to be settled, could have far-reaching effects on medical practice in the United States.

Provided due consideration is given to all factors previously mentioned, and that an indication for therapy does exist in a fully informed patient without any contraindications, the physician is justified in prescribing hormones.

Physicians should protect their rights through their own professional organizations and beware of inroads by uninformed, emotive lay groups in which they have no voice, which regrettably also often means governmental agencies. The objectives of organizations such as the FDA to reduce overuse and misuse of potent hormones are correct; there has to be some way, however, of presenting information to the public in a manner that is less frightening.

SPECIAL CLINICAL PROBLEMS

Fate of the Ovaries at Hysterectomy

From a preventive medicine standpoint, premature menopause and some of its consequent problems may be prevented by a more conservative attitude to ovaries at the time of surgery in premenopausal women. This applies, in particular, to the common procedure of bilateral ovariectomy during total abdominal hysterectomy in women before menopause.

The surgical removal of normal ovaries at the time of routine abdominal hysterectomy performed for benign conditions is a controversial subject in modern gynecology (Chapter 1). The incidence of surgical removal of ovaries at this time varies according to current practices in different gynecologic units and is poorly documented. Randall and Paloucek, for example, reported that no generally accepted criteria for ovarian preservation or indication for ovarian removal had been observed in one geographic area during the 25-year period reviewed.[20]

REASONS FOR REMOVAL OF OVARIES   There are three frequently cited reasons for surgical removal of normal ovaries:

Risk of Cancer in Retained Ovaries   The risk of subsequent development of carcinoma in retained ovaries following hysterectomy is generally considered to be small. Schabort, reviewing reasons for retaining ovaries, reported the incidence to be approximately 2 in 5000 hysterectomies.[21] However, Bloom found that 15 (10.6 percent) of 141 cases of primary adenocarcinoma of the ovary had previously had a hysterectomy or other pelvic operation performed. In 5 of these cases (3.5 percent) the ovaries had been conserved when the patient was over 50.[22] Counseller et al. reported on 1500 cases of proved carcinoma of the ovary of which 67 (4.5 percent) had undergone hysterectomy for a benign condition.[23] While 33 percent of these 67 patients were under 40 years of age, only 4.5 percent of these had ovarian carcinoma. The authors suggested that oophorectomy should therefore be performed only on patients over the age of 40. Unfortunately, even now it is difficult to define the absolute risk of subsequent development of carcinoma.

In summary, therefore, there are two ways in which to evaluate the problem. The first method is to determine the incidence of ovarian carcinoma in patients who have undergone previous hysterectomy. Experience in the last 25 years has shown this incidence to lie between 4 and 10 percent (Table 10-3). This method does not take into account the total number of hysterectomies with ovarian conservation that are not later complicated by ovarian cancer. The second approach, and the more valid one, is to follow up all such patients and to determine the overall incidence of ovarian cancer.[23A] The risk would then appear to be extremely low (Table 10-4).

There was a disturbing report that stilbestrol (DES) treatment for

Table 10–3.   The Incidence Of Previous Hysterectomy In Association with Current Admission For Ovarian Cancer.

Investigator	Year	Total number patients with ovarian cancer	Percentage with previous hysterectomy
Counseller et al.[23]	1955	1500	4.5
Fagan et al.[26]	1956	172	7.5
Bloom[22]	1962	141	10.6
Kaplan[41]	1977	142	10.5

Table 10–4. The Number And Percentage Of Patients Undergoing Hysterectomy With Conservation Of Ovaries And Later Developing Ovarian Cancer.

Investigator	Year	Number of Hysterectomies	Later Development of Ovarian Cancer	
			Number	Percent
Reycraft[23A]	1955	4500	9	0.2
Whitelaw[27]	1959	1215	0	0
Ranney[29]	1977	1557	4	0.25

menopausal symptoms might increase the risk of ovarian cancer,[24] but this conclusion was based on small numbers and a second study did not incriminate exogenous estrogens.[25]

To Avoid Ovarian Cysts or Pelvic Pain   There is no doubt that the conserved ovary after hysterectomy can in some cases cause pain or dyspareunia, or can become cystic and present as a persistent mass above the vaginal vault. This may give rise to anxiety on the part of the surgeon and patient, and lead to repeat surgery. The problem has been reported in as many as 5 percent of posthysterectomy patients.[21,26-28] Ranney and Abu-Ghazaleh, however, found that repeat surgery for benign indications was necessary in only 10 out of 1557 patients in whom ovarian tissue was retained at the time of hysterectomy, an incidence of less than 0.7 percent.[29]

Possible Loss of Function of Conserved Ovaries   The third common argument for routine removal of ovaries is the belief that following hysterectomy the ovaries soon become functionless. There is, however, evidence to show that the ovaries do continue to function from hysterectomy until the time of expected menopause.[29-33] Moreover, the fact that the postmenopausal ovary may also continue to function has been referred to previously.[31,34]

REASONS FOR CONSERVING OVARIES   The reasons for conserving ovaries have been more than adequately dealt with in the preceding chapters and can be itemized as follows:[30,35,36]

1. To prevent the development of postoperative menopausal symptoms (Chapter 7).
2. To prevent specific target organ regressive effects (Chapter 4).
3. To retard the development of osteoporosis (Chapter 5).
4. To delay if possible the onset of coronary heart disease (Chapter 6).
5. Psychologic reasons (Chapter 7). Simply stated, some women feel "incomplete" as females without their ovaries.[37]

CONCLUSION   What attitude should the gynecologic surgeon adopt toward ovaries of normal appearance at the time of hysterectomy? It is my affirmed opinion that the potential advantages of the functional ovary to the premenopausal woman far exceed the small risk of malignancy or subsequent benign pathology. I therefore believe strongly in conservation of ovaries of normal appearance in all women who are premenopausal at the time of surgery. After menopause the slight function of the residual ovary does not yet warrant its conservation, and the ovaries should be removed. This philosophy reaffirms the fact that it is the functional state of the ovary and not the chronological age of the patient that is of importance.

Abnormal Bleeding

POSTMENOPAUSAL BLEEDING   The dictum that postmenopausal bleeding indicates uterine cancer until proven otherwise remains the safest general principle to observe. Payne et al. reported a 17 percent incidence of cancer in patients with bleeding six to twelve months after menopause.[38] This disturbing report would suggest it wise to define postmenopausal bleeding as genital bleeding that occurs six months or more after menopause. Endometrial screening tests are described earlier in this chapter. Detailed physical examination, cytologic screening, and fractional dilation and curettage are generally indicated.

Reti et al. reported urinary estrogen values to correlate with the histologic appearance of the endometrium, being low when the endometrium was atrophic and highest when it was hyperplastic.[39] The origin of the estrogen appeared to be ovarian. Hormone assays are thus of potential value in the workup of the patient with postmenopausal bleeding.

The association between elevated circulating estrogen levels and endometrial histology also provides a theoretical foundation for the use of progestogens in the treatment of postmenopausal bleeding. Gambrell et al., for example, have recommended the use of progestogens for postmenopausal bleeding due to endometrial hyperplasia,[40] and reported that hyperplasia reverted to normal endometrium in 101 out of 105 treated patients. Hysterectomy was necessary in the remaining 4 patients. The use of progestogens is discussed in Chapter 9.

A problem does arise when there is a recurrence of postmenopausal bleeding in a patient in whom no pathologic cause for genital bleeding has been found. Kaplan reported 34 patients with recurrent postmenopausal bleeding, 32 of whom were treated by total abdominal hysterectomy and bilateral salpingo-oophorectomy.[41] Of the 34 patients, 4 were found to have carcinoma of the cervix and 5 had benign cystic glandular hyperplasia. He therefore recommended repeat cervical evaluation and dilatation and curettage in all such patients, and abdominal hysterectomy in obese patients in whom clinical evaluation was difficult.

BLEEDING RELATED TO HORMONE THERAPY   Any form of abnormal bleeding, be it unpredictable, prolonged, or excessive, requires histologic evaluation of the endometrium. This principle applies whether bleeding occurs on therapy (breakthrough bleeding) or during the pill-free days (withdrawal bleeding). In fact, a regular withdrawal response to estrogen is no guarantee of a healthy endometrium and all such patients should undergo an annual endometrial biopsy.[42] Moreover, routine endometrial biopsy not only aids diagnosis of early lesions which are amenable to definitive and completely corrective treatment, but can also uncover significant endometrial pathology before it becomes pathologic.[12]

Once a histologic diagnosis has been made and cancer excluded, there are two ways to treat abnormal bleeding responses to hormonal therapy. The first is to cease therapy and observe. The second is to adjust the type and dose of hormone being administered. In this respect, progestogens, alone or in combination with estrogen therapy, are drugs of considerable value. Bleeding can be regulated[42A] and a role in cancer prevention has been suggested.[40,42,43] The value of the progestogen is enhanced if it is given for longer than five days. Progestogen therapy for longer than seven days seems to induce unpleasant minor side effects (fluid retention, tender breasts, reversal of mental tonic effect). The author's personal preference, therefore, is to add progestogen to the final 7 days of a 25-day estrogen regime (Chapters 8,9).

Chronic Low Backache

Back pain is an almost universal symptom experienced by most people at some time. Women appear more prone to the problem than men because of hormonal influences, changes in posture during pregnancy, and the fact that gynecologic pathology may cause backache.

There is in fact an organic cause to nearly every complaint of backache.[44] The assessment of the severity of the pain, its cause, and the best treatment for the affected individual remains one of the more difficult problems in clinical medicine.

Chronic low backache in the peri- and postmenopausal woman may be related to osteoporosis and vertebral crush fracture (Chapter 5). However, there are other possible gynecologic causes. The pain usually results from involvement, or extension of the pathologic process into, the utero-sacral ligaments and is therefore sacral or lumbo-sacral in localization. The causes include chronic pelvic infection, severe utero-vaginal prolapse, and neoplasms. Gynecologic operations, particularly involving the dorso-lithotomy position, may also cause backache as the result of incorrect positioning or handling of the anesthetized patient.

Orthopedic causes of backache are numerous and may be due to mechanical factors or organic disease. Mechanical problems include intervertebral disc displacements, acute traumatic injuries, chronic postural strains, and spondylolisthesis. The pathologic syndromes include osteoporosis, osteoarthritis, acute chronic infections, and primary, and secondary neoplasms.

Correct treatment requires a correct diagnosis and the latter can often be elusive. The clinical evaluation of the more difficult cases is usually best accomplished by interconsultation between gynecologist, orthopedic surgeon, neurologist, and rheumatologist.

The postmenopausal patient suffering from incapacitating osteoporosis-induced backache can create a difficult therapeutic problem, the pain usually being relieved by bed rest and the immobilization itself exacerbating the problem. Intravenous calcium infusions can provide gratifying results in this situation, the pain often being relieved dramatically and the improvement lasting for three to six months. Calcium infusions of 15 mg/kg bodyweight are given intravenously in 1 liter of 5 percent dextrose water every 4 hours for 12 consecutive days. The procedure may need to be repeated at regular intervals.[45] The response to therapy is unexplained, but may be due to a hypercalcemic-induced reduction in nonautonomous subclinical hyperparathyroidism.

Headache

Headache is a symptom resulting from a large number of possible causes. No significant relationship has been demonstrated between the incidence of headache and menopause, or removal of ovaries.[46]

There does appear to be a definite relationship between oral contraceptive medication and the development of nonspecific headache.[46] The precise incidence is not known but seems to depend on the type of hormonal combination, and also to be in direct proportion to the dosage of hormones present in the pill, the lower-dosed pills being associated with a lower incidence of headache.

Most evidence favors the progestogenic component as the etiologic agent, but it would appear that some estrogen is necessary. The latter does not seem to have any direct causal relationship.

Any patients developing headache while on hormonal treatment after menopause should be investigated for coincidental causes. Even if excluded, hormonal therapy should probably be discontinued.

References

1.   Jacobs HS, Hull MGR, Murray MAF, Franks S: Therapy-oriented diagnosis of secondary amenorrhoea. Horm Res 6:268, 1975

2.   Black WP, Govan ADT: Laparoscopy and gonadal biopsy for assessment of gonadal function in primary amenorrhoea. Br Med J 1:672, 1972

3.   Evans JH: A review of 50 cases of primary amenorrhoea. Aust NZ J Obstet Gynaecol 11:7, 1971

4.   Kleinberg DL, Noel GL, Frantz AG: Galactorrhea. A study of 235 cases, including 48 with pituitary tumors. N Engl J Med 296:589, 1977

5.   Keye WR, Chang RJ, Jaffe RB: Prolactin secreting pituitary adenomas in women with amenorrhea or galactorrhea. Obstet Gynecol Surv 32:727, 1977

6.   Gilson MD, Knab DR: Primary amenorrhea. A simplified approach to diagnosis. Am J Obstet Gynecol 117:400, 1973

7.   Jewelewicz R: The diagnosis and treatment of amenorrheas. Fertil Steril 27:1347, 1976

8.   Donald RA, Baker DA, Metcalf MG, Turner ED: Assessment of ovarian function in perimenopausal women after stopping oral contraceptives. Br J Obstet Gynaecol 85:70, 1978

9.   Lauritzen C: Management of the patient at risk. Front Horm Res 5:230, 1978

10.   Vooijs GP: The morphology of endometrial proliferative reactions. Front Horm Res 5:76, 1978

11.   Jensen JA, Jensen JG: Vacuum curettage for diagnostic purposes. Ugeskr Laeger 130:2124, 1968

12.   Buchman MI, Kramer E, Feldman GB: Aspiration curettage for asymptomatic patients receiving estrogen. Obstet Gynecol 51:339, 1978

13.   Denis R, Barnett JM, Forbes SE: Diagnostic suction curettage. Obstet Gynecol 42:301, 1973

14.   Hutton JD, Morse AR, Anderson MC, Beard RW: Endometrial assessment with Isaacs cell sampler. Br Med J 1:947, 1978

15.   Reagan JW, Ng ABP: The Cells of Uterine Adenocarcinoma, 2nd ed. Basel, Karger, 1973

16.   Utian WH: Estrogen replacement in the menopause. In Wynn RM (ed): Obstetrics and Gynecology Annual, vol 8. New York, Appleton, 1979

17.   United States Food and Drug Administration: Estrogens and endometrial cancer. FDA Drug Bulletin, February/March 1976, p. 18

18.   Utian WH: The Menopause Manual. A Woman's Guide to the Menopause. Lancaster, MTP Press, 1979. Also published as Your Middle Years: A Doctor's Guide for Today's Woman. New York, Appleton, 1980

19.   Utian WH: Current status of menopause and postmenopausal estrogen therapy. Obstet Gynecol Surv 32:193, 1977

20.   Randall CL, Paloucek FP: The frequency of oophorectomy at the time of hysterectomy. Am J Obstet Gynecol 100:716, 1968

21.   Schabort JW: Oophorectomy—is wanton removal justified by fact? Trans Coll Phys Surg Gynaecol S Afr 4:11, 1960

22.   Bloom ML: Certain observations based on a study of 141 cases of primary adenocarcinoma of the ovaries. S Afr Med J 36:714, 1962

23.   Counseller VS, Hunt W, Haigler FH: Carcinoma of the ovary following hysterectomy. Am J Obstet Gynecol 69:538, 1955

23A.   Reycraft JL: Discussion on carcinoma of ovary following hysterectomy. Am J Obstet Gynecol 69:543, 1955

24.   Hoover R, Gray LA, Fraumeni JF: Stilboestrol (diethylstilbestrol) and the risk of ovarian cancer. Lancet 2:533, 1977

25.   Annegers JF, O'Fallon W, Kurland LT: Exogenous oestrogens and ovarian cancer. Lancet 2:869, 1977

26.   Fagan GE, Allen ED, Klawans AH: Ovarian neoplasms and repeat pelvic surgery. Obstet Gynecol 7:418, 1956

27.   Whitelaw RG: Ovarian activity following hysterectomy. J Obstet Gynaecol Br Cwlth 65:917, 1958

28.   Grogan RH, Duncan CJ: Ovarian salvage in routine abdominal hysterectomy. Am J Obstet Gynecol 70:1277, 1955

29.   Ranney B, Abu-Ghazaleh S: The future function and fortune of ovarian tissue which is retained in vivo during hysterectomy. Am J Obstet Gynecol 128:626, 1977

30.   Utian WH: Clinical and metabolic effects of the menopause and the role of replacement oestrogen therapy. Unpublished Ph.D. Thesis, University of Cape Town, 1970

31.   Procope BJ: Studies on the urinary excretion, biological effects, and origin of oestrogens in postmenopausal women. Acta Endocrinol [Suppl] (kbh) 60:135, 1968

32.   Beavis ELG, Brown JB, Smith MA: Ovarian function after hysterectomy with conservation of ovaries in premenopausal women. J Obstet Gynaecol Br Cwlth 76:969, 1969

33.   Beling CG, Marcus SL, Markham SM: Functional activity of the corpus luteum after hysterectomy. J Clin Endocrinol Metab 30:30, 1970

34.   Poliak A, Jones GES, Goldberg B, Solomon D, Woodruff JB: Effect of human chorionic gonadotropin on postmenopausal women. Am J Obstet Gynecol 101:731, 1968

35.   Johansson BW, Kaij L, Kullander S, et al.: On some late effects of bilateral oophorectomy in the age range 15-30 years. Acta Obstet Gynecol Scand 54:449, 1975

36.   Chakravarti S, Collins WP, Newton JR, Oram DH, Studd JWW: Endocrine changes and symptomatology after oophorectomy in premenopausal women. Br J Obstet Gynaecol 84:769, 1977

37.   Murless BC: The fate of the ovaries at hysterectomy. S Afr J Obstet Gynaecol 2:62, 1964

38.   Payne FL, Wright RC, Fetterman HH: Postmenopausal bleeding. Am J Obstet Gynecol 77:1216, 1959

39.   Reti LL, Rome RM, Brown JB, Fortune DW: Urinary oestrogen and pregnanediol excretion, endometrial and ovarian pathology and body weight in women with postmenopausal bleeding. Br J Obstet Gynaecol 85:857, 1978

40.   Gambrell RD, Castaneda TA, Ricci CA: Management of postmenopausal bleeding to prevent endometrial cancer. Maturitas 1:99, 1978

41.   Kaplan E: Recurrent postmenopausal bleeding. S Afr Med J 52:1121, 1977

42.   Sturdee DW, Wade-Evans T, Paterson MEL, Thom M, Studd JWW: Relations between bleeding pattern, endometrial histology, and oestrogen treatment in menopausal women. Br Med J 1:1575, 1978

42A.   Whitehead MI: The effects of oestrogens and progestogens on the post-menopausal endometrium. Maturitas 1:87, 1978

43.   Gambrell RD: The prevention of endometrial cancer in postmenopausal women with progestogens. Maturitas 1:107, 1978

44.   Adler M, Utian WH: Chronic low backache in the middle-aged woman. S Afr J Physiotherapy 22:5, 1970

45.   Epstein S: Metabolic bone disease — recent developments. S Afr Med J 48:350, 1974

46.   Utian WH: Oestrogen, headache and oral contraceptives. S Afr Med J 48:2105, 1974

11
The Future

Thucydides (c. 460-400 BCE) expressed a sentiment long ago that best mirrors my hope for this book: "I shall be content if it is judged useful by those inquirers who desire an exact knowledge of the past as an aid to the interpretation of the future, which in the course of human things must resemble if it does not reflect it."

The exhaustive and exhausting search of the literature that preceded the writing of this monograph has been illuminating for several reasons beyond the obvious. Perhaps most striking of all is the amount of reduplicated and often ill-directed effort. Repeatedly, even in the most recent literature, authors pointedly ignore or appear unaware of previous accomplishments, and make claims for "firsts" in medicine. Regrettably, and all too often, there is a failure to build properly on existing foundations and errors in study design recur again and again.

Equally unfortunate is the tendency of some authors to become "champions" of estrogen therapy, and to write pseudoscientific communications that read like drug testimonials. This misdirected enthusiasm is almost unique to the estrogen-replacement therapy literature. Inevitably, a substantial number of these papers fail as scientific communications because they are more obviously written to prove a pet theory or drive home a point than to impartially evaluate the results of a suitably tested hypothesis. I cannot help but be reminded by these antics of Santayana's definition of a fanatic—the person who redoubles his efforts when he has forgotten his aim.

The present and the past have been dealt with in depth, and inevitably become history. What of the future? There is much reason to be confident. The dramatic increase in sound scientific investigation during the last decade bears witness to this, and provides hope for what is to come. Climacteric-related events are being increasingly well defined. Advances in knowledge are escalating in all disciplines. Mistakes of the past have been recognized. Well-planned prospective evaluations of normal physiologic events, pathologic changes, and drug responses are in progress or are being initiated.

Investigators, as individuals or groups in research centers, have become more aware of each other and of the work that is being accomplished. Instrumental in this development has been the dramatic expansion of information storage and retrieval systems. Of greater significance, to my mind, has been the reduction in the size of the globe. Simplification of travel, and the willingness to do so, has resulted in researchers from all over the world getting together at meetings ranging from small group workshops to international menopause conferences. Fortunately, scientific respect and cooperation supersede political barriers. The growth of this tendency is to be encouraged.

A few specific developments likely to be seen in the near future include:

1. Precise structural and chemical effects of altered hormone profiles on specific target tissues will be even better defined. Coincidental aging features will be better differentiated and explained. Moreover, hormone receptor mechanisms and their influence on protein synthesis will be clarified.

2. The specific causative mechanism of the hot flush will be described. This is likely to involve a prostaglandin-related pathway. This should allow for the development and introduction of nonhormonal drugs including antiprostaglandins that will inhibit the sporadic triggering of this disturbing symptom.

3. The currently available steroidal hormones will undergo escalating pharmacokinetic scrutiny for harmful and beneficial effects, and their exact therapeutic indications will be further clarified.

4. Combinations of hormones, including nonsex hormones (e.g., thyroid, parathyroid) will be clinically evaluated for synergistic and antagonistic properties.

5. There is distinct promise that new hormone analogues and antagonists will be developed with properties more specific to one or another metabolic process. Agencies such as the FDA, however, will delay the introduction of such substances into clinical use for many years. This cautionary attitude is justifiable in light of previous irresponsible estrogen use, but, hopefully, the regulatory hurdles will not be made insurmountable and counterproductive. Discretion is urged upon clinicians, investigators, and the regulatory bodies themselves.

6. The route of administration of steroidal hormones will receive increasing attention. Percutaneous routes in particular, by avoidance of the first liver passage and consequent alteration of metabolic pathways, may result in reduced toxic effects.

7. Psycho-neuro-endocrine physiology will continue to develop as a major research area, and clarification of, for example, catecholestrogen metabolism is likely to have a high yeild in terms of explanation and treatment of behavioral phenomena such as depression and anxiety.

8. Less abuse of estrogen therapy, with stricter observation of basic physiologic principles and use of selected progestogens, is likely to manifest in declining uterine cancer rates.

9. The key to the puzzling interrelationships between cholesterol and lipid metabolism, coronary heart disease, and gallstone production

may open the door to explaining the cause of these problems and to eventual effective prevention programs.

10. A better understanding of menopause-related events by physicians will flow over into improved educational programs in the general population and, specifically, in better-informed patients. Hopefully, this will also witness a positive change in attitude by society toward menopause and aging, with an ultimate decrease in the psycho-socio-cultural contribution to symptom formation.

These and more are the prospects for the future. Untoward effects of the climacteric as well as the therapeutic modalities, as yet unconsidered, may also be revealed. It therefore behooves all parties interested in the health care of women in their middle years to keep an open and questioning mind, to accept developments where proven, and to avoid dogma and prejudice: "We should all be concerned about the future because we will all have to spend the rest of our lives there." (C.F. Kettering 1876-1958)

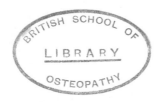

Index